Advance Praise for *The Way Out*

"*The Way Out* offers a wonderfully clear and compelling combination of personal experience and the latest breakthroughs in brain science to show how to reduce chronic pain. Beautifully written, with gentle humor and genuine compassion, the authors start from acknowledging the reality of chronic pain and invite you to try techniques that promise a new freedom that might have seemed impossible—a transformation that will affect both you and those with whom you share your life."

—MARK WILLIAMS, PROFESSOR EMERITUS OF
CLINICAL PSYCHOLOGY, UNIVERSITY OF OXFORD,
AND COAUTHOR OF *MINDFULNESS*

"If you suffer from chronic pain (or know someone who does), *The Way Out* is an optimistic, science-based book about managing the mind-body connection to healing. Alan Gordon writes with compassion, empathy, and a deep understanding of living with pain. Finding relief from his own suffering prompted him to find freedom for others."

—SHARON SALZBERG, AUTHOR OF
LOVINGKINDNESS AND *REAL CHANGE*

"*The Way Out* highlights the role of neuroplasticity in chronic pain and explores how to tackle it. This is a great positive step forward in chronic pain treatment."

—CLIFFORD WOOLF, MD, PROFESSOR OF NEUROLOGY AND
NEUROBIOLOGY, HARVARD MEDICAL SCHOOL

"The strain in pain lies mainly in the brain. This accessible, warm book is a reminder of how you can learn to better control pain by learning to think differently about it."

"It's long been assumed that chronic pain is irreversible, but *The Way Out* introduces an approach that proves otherwise. I have seen the power of this treatment firsthand. Patients who suffered for years or even decades have made remarkable recoveries. *The Way Out* is, quite simply, the most effective treatment for chronic pain."

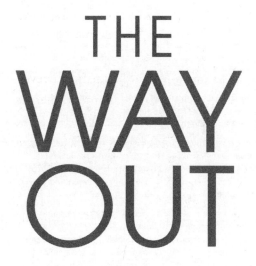

THE
WAY
OUT

A Revolutionary,
Scientifically Proven Approach
to Healing Chronic Pain

ALAN GORDON AND **ALON ZIV**

Avery
an imprint of Penguin Random House
New York

AVERY

an imprint of Penguin Random House LLC
penguinrandomhouse.com

Library of Congress Cataloging-in-Publication Data
Names: Gordon, Alan (Psychotherapist), author. | Ziv, Alon, author.
Title: The way out : a revolutionary, scientifically proven approach to healing chronic
pain / Alan Gordon and Alon Ziv.
Description: New York : Avery, 2021. | Includes index.
Identifiers: LCCN 2020020094 (print) | LCCN 2020020095 (ebook) |
ISBN 9780593086834 (hardcover) | ISBN 9780593086841 (ebook)
Subjects: LCSH: Chronic pain—Alternative treatment. |
Pain—Psychological aspects. | Mind and body therapies.
Classification: LCC RB127 .G66 2021 (print) | LCC RB127 (ebook) |
DDC 616/.0472—dc23
LC record available at https://lccn.loc.gov/2020020094
LC ebook record available at https://lccn.loc.gov/2020020095
p.   cm.

Printed in the United States of America
1st Printing

Book design by Lorie Pagnozzi

To Christie,
For your friendship, collaboration, and the countless
pictures of your dog sleeping in a shoe.

A.G.

To Krystal,
As long as we're together, life will always be good.

A.Z.

contents

foreword

I didn't start out as a believer. Like many people, I was uncertain about how deeply mind-body interventions can affect the course of chronic pain, and for whom. I am inherently skeptical. But I also really want to know the answers, so my instinct is to gather scientific evidence. I have spent a good part of my career studying whether changing your mind can affect your brain and body. If it can, which kinds of changes are possible, and which are not? What conditions are required to make these changes? If your thoughts do affect your body, are they large enough to be meaningful, and profound enough to last?

When I first met Alan Gordon, my overwhelming experience of him was that he *is* a believer. As a former chronic pain sufferer who has now recovered, he believes that it is possible to go from suffering from debilitating pain to being pain-free, without drugs or surgery. He demonstrates that belief in action with an infectious enthusiasm and a commitment to helping each individual he works with. Over the past two years, I've experienced a transformation in my belief as well. I've come to believe that the right ideas about chronic pain, put into practice through mind-body treatment, can have dramatic benefits for many or even most people—even after real injuries that give rise to real pain.

I got involved with Alan via serendipity. I had met Alan's colleague, Dr. Howard Schubiner, several times at scientific meetings. I'm a neuroscientist studying pain circuitry with functional magnetic resonance imaging (fMRI). I remember Howard telling me, "We have this treatment that really works. We've been helping people recover from chronic pain for years—you should study that!" It didn't click. I'm fascinated by mind-body interventions, but we were studying basic brain circuits, with no funding or infrastructure to study patients.

My graduate student Yoni Ashar and I had been brainstorming topics for his Ph.D. dissertation. Yoni suffered from chronic back pain for several years, which made back pain a personally meaningful topic of study. This is where the serendipity begins. Howard got in touch again, with fMRI imaging results from a patient who showed dramatic improvement after Alan's treatment. The results were tantalizing. They showed changes in the medial prefrontal cortex and the anterior insula. These areas of the brain are connected, and part of a network that assigns personal meaning to input that comes from the body. These areas have also been among the most frequently identified in studies of chronic pain. It seems as if part of the problem for many people with chronic pain is the *significance* the brain attaches to pain and things that might cause it. We decided to go for it and start a study on Alan's treatment in people with chronic back pain.

We started with modest goals. At first, we planned to scan just a few people undergoing treatment. Then Yoni attended Alan and Howard's weekend training course and saw the power of the treatment in action. Meanwhile, Alan started a crowd-funding campaign that generated both money for the study and, even more important, excitement from people who really wanted this to happen. I found some additional grant funding, and we expanded the study even further. We ended up conducting one of the largest fMRI studies of back pain to date. We did this with about a quarter of the funding that it would typically take, because everyone—Yoni, Alan, Howard, and our terrific research assistants Laurie Polisky, Zach Anderson, and others—believed in the importance of this project and put their hearts and souls into getting it done.

The results of our study are what turned me into a believer. After being in chronic pain for, on average, eleven years, the majority of patients were pain-free or nearly so after a month of treatment. And so far, they appear to be staying that way. Let me be clear that there are still many questions to answer: For which kinds of pain, and which kinds of people, are such results possible? What are the "active ingredients," and how much does improvement depend on who is delivering the treatment? How strongly does improvement depend on a patient's openness to being "cured"? Chronic pain has multiple causes in the body and brain. We do not yet understand these, and we simply cannot measure pathology well enough in humans to determine the best treatment for every individual. But we did our best to make our study a rigorous, objective, unbiased test of how well Alan's treatment works—and the data showed that people got better.

Even more interesting is what this study, and others, tells us about chronic pain. This is a spectacular time for the neuroscience of pain, with studies demonstrating unequivocally that injury produces changes in the nervous system at multiple levels: in the body, in the spinal cord, and in the brain. Higher-level brain centers associated with mood, memory, and long-term planning can block pain or enhance it, drive recovery or make pain chronic. In humans, those higher-level centers create our personality, our emotions, and our sense of who we are and where we belong in the world. So, in a very real way, chronic pain is entangled with our understanding of what the pain means to us and our outlook for the future. This does not mean that pain is not "real." Pain can have real causes in the body, spinal cord, and brain and still be treated with a mind-body approach, because all these levels are connected.

The neuroscience of pain has demonstrated that the causes of chronic pain may be different from the causes of acute pain after injury, and may in many cases reside in the brain. Mind-body treatment can help us understand what kinds of movements and activities are okay, even in the presence of pain, which in turn can help our brains "unlearn" chronic pain.

What is remarkable about Alan's treatment in particular is that information is a large part of the cure. New information can change our beliefs about the causes of pain and the narratives we tell ourselves about it. Often this change can take work and practice, but it can also happen suddenly, in a flash of insight. I've witnessed this personally. One member of my lab had shoulder pain for several years, and seems to have been cured after hearing about these techniques. Another friend and colleague, through talking with Yoni about our research, also came to a new understanding about her chronic pain. She experienced a dramatic healing and told me that this transformation saved her life.

In the book *How to Know God*, Swami Prabhavananda and Christopher Isherwood distinguish between different kinds of beliefs. One kind of belief is faith. With faith, we must believe in the absence of, or in spite of, evidence provided by our own senses. The second kind is provisional belief. When learning to meditate, they point out, one must believe in its benefits only enough to give it a try. It is this second kind of belief that I urge you to adopt. You don't have to have faith that chronic pain can be cured; you just have to believe enough to start working with the ideas in this book with an open mind. Try it and see what happens.

–Tor Wager
Distinguished Professor of Neuroscience
Dartmouth College

CHAPTER 1

This Kid's Brain Could Change the World

"He's in a ton of pain. His parents are desperate. Do you think you can help?"

It was December 2016, and I'd just received a call from CBS's *The Doctors*, a long-running medical talk show produced by Dr. Phil. For this particular episode, they were trying to help Casey, a sixteen-year-old with chronic abdominal pain so severe that it would regularly cause him to pass out. Casey's doctors were baffled.

As the director of the Pain Psychology Center in Los Angeles, I specialize in treating chronic pain and other physical symptoms. The producer on the phone wanted to know if my team and I might be able to help poor Casey with his pain.

Two years before, Casey was a run-of-the-mill ninth grader at John Burroughs High School in Burbank, California. He loved baseball and *Star Wars*; he hated algebra and chemistry. He seemed on track for your standard high school experience—until about three months into his freshman year, when he felt a stabbing pain in his stomach.

Thinking it might be appendicitis, his parents rushed him to the hospital. But the doctors couldn't find anything wrong. Months passed and his pain persisted. They got every test imaginable—MRIs, CT scans, exploratory surgeries—but everything came back negative.

Casey, in the meantime, was finding it harder and harder to function. He quit the baseball team and eventually had to drop out of school. Casey's long, painful journey finally led him to *The Doctors*, and then they called me.

"We'll need to look over his medical records," I said, "but I think there's a good chance we can help."

"Great," the producer said. "One more thing: Is there anything we can do for the episode to show the effect of getting out of pain?"

She made a good point. This was going to be on TV. They needed something visual for the viewers at home. How could we show Casey's pain, something that he experiences internally?

I thought about it for a moment and said, "Maybe we can get an fMRI of his brain before and after treatment?"

Functional magnetic resonance imaging, or fMRI, is a scan that shows brain activity. I thought it would be interesting to see how Casey's brain might change once he was out of pain. I didn't know it at the time, but that casual suggestion would lead to one of the most groundbreaking studies in the history of pain.

But to really tell you the story of Casey's pain, I first need to tell you about my own.

Me, My Chair, and My Mom

In my mid-twenties, life was good. I was in graduate school for psychotherapy at USC. I was an outgoing, active guy. I hung out with my friends. I went to Dodgers games. I was in a kickball league (my team even made it to Nationals!). But during my second year of grad school, everything changed. I developed severe lower back pain, and it completely derailed my life.

Even something as simple as sitting through a movie became a two-hour-long nightmare. Dodgers games were out of the question. I couldn't watch sports, let alone play them. The stiff classroom seats at USC caused me so much pain, I had to buy a soft, lean-back chair from Office Depot and roll it from class to class. In case you're wondering, lugging a giant chair everywhere you go is not great for your social life.

I saw three of the leading back specialists in Los Angeles. One of them told me that my pain was caused by a disc herniation. One of them told me that my symptoms were due to disc degeneration. One of them told me that my back hurt because I was just too tall.

I couldn't make myself shorter, but I tried every other treatment imaginable: physical therapy, biofeedback, acupuncture, acupressure. Nothing helped. I got so many MRI scans of my back, my friends joked that my spine was turning into a magnet.

After about six months, I got an epidural injection. It didn't cure me, but it cut my pain in half. Life was once again bearable . . . for about eight days. Until one morning, out of nowhere, I felt like a grenade went off in my head. It was the most excruciating headache I'd ever had.

And it stayed.

Chronic daily headache, the internet told me, had no known cause and no known cure. Terrific.

After seeing even more doctors, I found a headache specialist who diagnosed me with high cerebrospinal fluid (CSF) pressure. He prescribed some medication, which didn't help.

Here's the thing about high-CSF-pressure headaches: the pain is worse when you lie down. So I couldn't sit up because it hurt my back, and I couldn't lie down because it hurt my head. My father, practical man that he is, suggested that I try to find a way to live at a forty-five-degree angle. Thanks, Dad.

Over the next several years, I developed the following additional symptoms:

- upper back pain
- neck pain
- shoulder pain
- knee pain
- heel pain
- tongue pain (who gets tongue pain?)
- eye pain
- tooth pain
- toe pain (three different toes!)
- hip pain
- stomach pain
- wrist pain
- foot pain
- leg pain
- TMJ
- heartburn
- vertigo
- tinnitus
- itching
- fatigue

In short, I was a mess. Doctors were scared of me. I had plenty of diagnoses to go along with these symptoms: bulging discs, partially torn rotator cuff, repetitive strain injury, etc. But none of the medical treatments helped me.

Pain took over my life. It was too hard to put on a happy face with my friends, so I withdrew socially. I couldn't work. I put my life completely on hold to try to deal with my pain. I even moved back home with my parents.

One day my mom gave me a book about a mind-body approach to treating pain. She told me that her friend's son had read it, and it had helped him get rid of his back pain. She's a loving mother, and she was trying to help me. So I did what any rational chronic pain sufferer would do. I threw the book across the room.

"A book isn't going to help me, Mom. The pain isn't in my head. I have a bunch of diagnoses from doctors."

She shrugged and left the room. You don't argue with someone in chronic pain.

A year later I finally read the book, and I spoke with my mom's friend's son. The book didn't get rid of my pain, but it opened my mind to the possibility that I could. It was an important first step. I decided to learn everything there is to know about pain.

I studied the neuroscience of pain. I learned that pain involves both the body and the brain. Normally, the brain gets signals from throughout the body and processes them. If the body experiences an injury, the brain generates the feeling of pain.

But sometimes the system goes haywire. Sometimes the "pain switch" in our brains can get stuck in the on position and cause chronic pain.

We call this neuroplastic pain. Normal pain is caused by damage to the body. But pain that persists after an injury has healed, or pain that has no clear physical cause, is usually neuroplastic pain. In chapter 2, I'll explain why neuroplastic pain develops and how to determine if you have it.

I realized that I was suffering from neuroplastic pain. I'd been focused on fixing my body, but to get rid of my pain, I needed to target my brain. The mind-body approach to chronic pain was relatively new, and the treatments were underdeveloped. So I created new techniques to rewire my brain and restore the natural order.

I still have bulging discs. I still have high cerebrospinal fluid pressure. I probably still have a partially torn rotator cuff. But I don't have any pain. I eliminated all twenty-two of my symptoms.

Along the way, I realized that I wasn't alone. In fact, we're in the midst of a chronic pain epidemic. More than 50 million adults suffer from chronic pain in the United States alone. Globally, the number is estimated to be 1.2 billion!

Treating chronic pain became my life's work. I founded the Pain Psychology Center and began helping other sufferers. In my experience, the majority of chronic pain is neuroplastic pain. Over the years, we've refined our techniques into a consistently effective system—Pain Reprocessing Therapy—and we've helped people overcome every form of pain imaginable.

And every patient that my team and I treat, no matter where their pain is or how long they've endured it, asks the same question:

The Conversation

Patient: Are you saying my pain isn't real?

Me: Well, do you feel it?

Patient: Yes.

Me: Does it hurt?

Patient: Yes.

Me: Then it's real.

I've always found it bizarre that some pain is considered real while other pain isn't.

When I was a student at UCLA, my fraternity once had a hypnotist come to a rush-week event. My buddy Jamie volunteered to get hypnotized. This clearly unethical hypnotist put Jamie in a trance and told him that his arm was on fire. Jamie ran around frantically and dunked his arm in an ice chest. It was hilarious.

I asked Jamie afterward if it had hurt. "It was the worst pain I've ever felt," he said (with some choice swear words). How could that be?

A study at the University of Pittsburgh looked into hypnosis and pain. Researchers placed subjects in an fMRI machine and administered pain with a hot probe. The pain regions of the participants' brains lit up clear as day. Then the scientists took the same subjects, hypnotized them, and induced pain through suggestion. The exact same areas of their brains lit up on the fMRIs. Whether the pain was induced physically or through hypnosis, the sensation was the same as far as the brain was concerned.

Pain is pain, and it is always real. And because all pain is processed in the brain, our brains have extraordinary power to affect where, when, and how much pain we experience.

Our Aching Backs

Back pain is the most common form of chronic pain and the leading cause of disability worldwide. If you suffer from chronic back pain, you may have had some version of this conversation:

> **You:** I've had back pain for three months. It hurts when I sit, it hurts when I stand, and it hurts when I walk.

> **Orthopedic doctor:** Hmm, an MRI of your spine shows that you have a four-millimeter disc herniation at L2-L3 with partial nerve root compression.

> **You:**

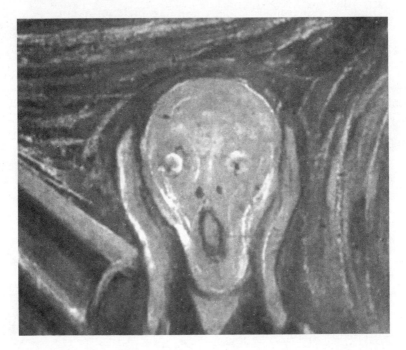

The diagnosis makes it sound like your poor, defective spine has an enormous disc jutting out and crushing one of your nerves. The image is terrifying, but also somehow appealing—you have pain in your back, and the doctor found a problem there. All you have to do is fix the problem in your back, and the pain will go away, right?

Sadly, no. Studies have shown that many of the most common back surgeries are simply not effective. In fact, continued back pain after surgery is so common that there's even a name for it: failed back surgery syndrome.

Here's the reality: Most of us have disc bulges or herniations. Most of us have disc degeneration and arthritis. You know who has perfectly unblemished spines? Babies. Their discs are all wonderfully plump, and their adorable little joints are completely free from inflammation. As we go through life, we develop wear and tear. This deterioration of our body is natural and inevitable. A study in the *New England Journal of Medicine* found that 64 percent of people with no back pain have disc bulges, protrusions, herniations, or disc degeneration. These structural changes are actually quite normal and usually unrelated to pain.

Even when there are findings on an MRI, they usually don't line up with the physical symptoms. A Swiss study recruited people with chronic back pain and looked for things like disc degeneration and bulging discs. The scientists found that there was no relationship between any of these structural issues and the subjects' symptoms.

So, if structural damage isn't responsible for most cases of chronic back pain, what is?

Combining cutting-edge neuroscience with a little bit of

Nostradamus, a group of scientists at Northwestern University embarked on a new frontier: predicting pain. These researchers tracked patients after an initial episode of back pain and tried to predict who would go on to develop chronic pain. Amazingly, their predictions were accurate 85 percent of the time.

The scientists didn't conduct any back exams. They didn't look at X-rays or MRIs of the spines. In fact, they didn't look at the patients' backs at all; they looked only at their brains. By taking brain scans and looking at the level of connectivity between two key areas, the researchers were able to determine with a high level of accuracy whose pain would persist and whose would resolve.

Most cases of chronic back pain are not caused by structural damage to the spine. The pain is 100 percent real, but it's neuroplastic pain. To treat it, we need to target the brain, not the body.

Real Whiplashes and Fake Car Crashes

Imagine you're driving. You pull up to a red light, and as you come to a stop, you hear the sound of screeching brakes. You look in the rearview mirror just in time to see the driver behind you, cell phone in hand, with a look of horror in his eyes. You brace. At the moment of impact, your head snaps back and then forward. Ouch. This is called whiplash, and it often leads to head or neck pain. Whiplash is a type of neck sprain, and as with other sprains, with a little rest, it should heal completely in a few days.

But sometimes the whiplash pain doesn't heal. When an injury of this kind persists, it's referred to as chronic whiplash syndrome. In many countries, this syndrome has become an epidemic, with up to 10 percent of accident victims becoming permanently disabled.

The strange thing is, studies have shown that there's no structural basis for chronic whiplash syndrome. In other words, the body heals, but for some reason, the pain persists.

A group of researchers thought the answer to this medical mystery might be found in the far reaches of northern Europe. Lithuania is a small country on the Baltic Sea known for beautiful scenery and great basketball teams (it's the national sport). But one thing you won't find in Lithuania is chronic whiplash. They have cars, they have roads, and they have rear-end collisions, but no persistent neck pain.

The scientists evaluated hundreds of rear-end-collision victims and followed their recovery. Many of the victims had neck pain immediately after the accident. But one year later, their symptoms were no different from members of the general population. Chronic whiplash simply doesn't exist in Lithuania.

But if car accidents don't cause chronic whiplash, what does?

Researchers in Germany conducted a brilliant and slightly crazy experiment to find out. They recruited volunteers for a car-crash study. The participants were placed in the driver's seat of one car and slammed from behind by another car. Except they weren't, actually. The whole thing was fake. Or as the scientists call it, a "placebo collision."

How do you fake a car accident? The researchers smashed a bottle to simulate the sound of a crash, and through a complicated set of pulleys and a ramp, the test subjects' car moved forward slightly. There was no actual contact from the other car, but the participants thought they had been rear-ended. The sneaky scientists even scattered broken glass on the ground to further make it seem like the car had been hit.

Three days after the fake collision, 20 percent of the participants had neck pain. Four weeks later, 10 percent of them still had symptoms. Their pain was real, but there was no structural damage to their bodies. There couldn't have been, because there was no actual impact to the car.

The pain didn't come from the participants' necks but from something in their brains: belief. They believed that they had been in a collision, and they believed that chronic whiplash was a possible side effect. The Lithuanians didn't share that belief. Because chronic whiplash isn't a phenomenon in their country, it didn't even occur to the car crash victims in Lithuania that their pain could persist. So it didn't.

Why would believing in chronic whiplash lead to actual chronic whiplash? The answer to that is in chapter 3, but for now it's clear that our brains are powerful and complex enough to generate and maintain pain. It's counterintuitive because the pain feels like it's coming from our bodies, but it's neuroplastic pain, and it's coming from our brains. That's actually good news though, because if your brain can give you pain, it can also take it away.

Back pain and whiplash are just a couple of chronic conditions often caused by neuroplastic pain. I have stories and studies about so many more, including headaches, stomach pain, pelvic pain, joint pain, nerve pain, irritable bowel syndrome, and repetitive strain injury. I won't go into the details of each one, but my team and I have successfully treated all of them with Pain Reprocessing Therapy.

In each case, patients experience physical symptoms, but physical treatments don't help. By targeting the brain instead of the body, patients can finally get relief from their pain.

Which brings us back to Casey, my abdominal-pain patient from *The Doctors.*

Casey's Cure

Casey and his family sat in my office, trying to ignore the two cameramen several feet away. Casey's mom, fighting back tears, told me their story. She said, "We've tried everything. Medication, procedures, surgeries . . . Nothing's worked."

I explained to Casey the phenomenon of neuroplastic pain—how our brains can generate very real pain even in the absence of injury, and how this pain is reversible. Casey allowed himself to feel a glimmer of hope, and tears streamed down his face.

"We're gonna fix it, buddy," his mom said, trying hard to believe her own words.

Casey and I met weekly. We talked about how his pain had developed and why it persisted. I taught him the elements of Pain Reprocessing Therapy, and we practiced them together. After four weeks, he was swinging a baseball bat in my office with no pain. At six weeks, he was running up and down the halls at full speed (much to the surprise of my officemates). After three months, he was pain-free.

Soon after, he was back in school, where he belonged. And playing center field on the baseball team!

Per the request of *The Doctors*, we got an fMRI of Casey's brain both before and after treatment. The medical literature is full of fMRIs of people experiencing various degrees of pain. But no one had ever studied what the brain looks like when chronic pain is cured. Would there be visible changes in Casey's brain?

A few days later, I got a call from the radiologist who conducted Casey's fMRIs. "This is incredible," he said. "The difference between the two images is staggering." He sent me the scans right away.

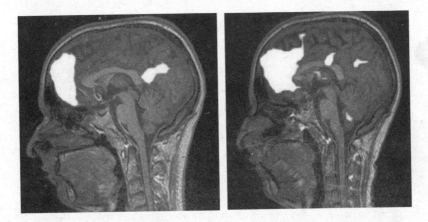

Casey's brain activity before treatment (left) and after treatment (right)

On the whim of a daytime talk show, we found ourselves with the first fMRI case study for eliminating chronic pain. As I looked at the dramatic differences in Casey's before and after scans, I thought to myself, "This kid's brain could change the world."

A New Understanding of Pain

Casey's scans were remarkable. There were changes in the medial prefrontal cortex, the nucleus accumbens, and the anterior insula. These regions of the brain have two things in common: they all sound like spells from Harry Potter and they're all involved in processing pain.

Casey's results were tantalizing, but he was just a single case study. Were the changes a fluke or did Pain Reprocessing Therapy actually rewire Casey's brain? We knew there was just one person to reach out to: world-famous neuroscientist Tor Wager. Over the past ten years, there has been a revolution in our understanding of pain, and Tor Wager has been at the forefront.

For centuries, scientists have looked at the brain as something of a black box. We knew the basics: it receives signals from the body, it generates thoughts and feelings, and sometimes it'll freeze when we eat ice cream too fast. We even had a rough idea of which areas of the brain did what. But mostly we knew that it was a very important, pinkish-gray blob.

But fMRI technology changed all that. Thanks to fMRIs like Casey's, we can see exactly which parts of the brain are being used in different situations. For the first time, we have a front-row view of this complex system, and it's given us a whole new understanding of pain. Over the past decade, thousands of fMRI studies have been done on different aspects of pain. While there is still a lot to learn, we've made two major discoveries.

First, it's become clear that chronic pain is completely different from short-term pain. It acts differently, responds to treatment differently, and even involves different parts of the brain. I'll talk about this more in chapter 2.

Second, pain is much more complicated than we originally thought. There isn't just one "pain center" of the brain; fMRI studies have found that multiple areas of the brain are associated with pain. And when I say "multiple," I mean *multiple*.

This brings us back to Tor Wager, who showed just how complicated pain is. Dr. Wager used artificial intelligence to analyze thousands of brain scans. He discovered a unique pattern of brain activity when people experience pain. This "pain signature" involves forty-four different parts of the brain. Forty-four! Half of these brain regions are involved in increasing pain, and the other half in decreasing it.

Clearly, the brain does some very complex processing to generate pain, and no one understands it better than Tor Wager. We immediately sent him Casey's fMRIs. And he responded with an incredible opportunity.

The Boulder Back Pain Study

As luck would have it, Dr. Wager was about to start a new study on chronic back pain, and all the participants were going to get fMRIs of their brains before and after treatment.

Dr. Wager was impressed with Casey's results, and he offered to add another group to the study using our treatment. The good news was that a randomized controlled study with a world-renowned neuroscientist could give Pain Reprocessing Therapy some serious scientific credibility. The bad news was that Dr. Wager's lab was at the University of Colorado Boulder, a thousand miles from Los Angeles.

We jumped at the chance.

The next year of my life was a whirlwind of travel. I helped run the Boulder Back Pain Study while still treating my patients back in Los Angeles and teaching at USC. I took four flights a week. Every week. In the process, I accumulated enough frequent-flier miles to go halfway to the moon.

The study team was incredible. In addition to Dr. Wager, there were Zack, Laurie, and Judith, who ran the brain scans. Dr. Howard Schubiner did the medical consultations. And then there was the man who ran the show: Yoni, a thirty-two-year-old wunderkind with the mind of Aristotle and the effortless cool of James Dean. Yoni and I had a great working relationship. He was the practical one. I was more . . . idealistic.

Yoni: We need to define our study goals before we start so it's completely objective.

Me: Great.

Yoni: Every week we'll have the participants fill out the BPI [the Brief Pain Inventory is a standard form for reporting pain levels on a scale of 0–10]. Then we'll compare their scores at the beginning and end of the treatment to see if their pain is reduced.

Me: I don't want to just reduce their pain. I want to cure them.

Yoni: Well, chronic pain studies don't really report statistics on "curing," because patients are rarely cured. The standard is to just try to reduce their pain levels.

Me: We're going to cure them.

Yoni: Okay . . .

Yoni was skeptical (Yoni is always skeptical), but he agreed. If a patient's average pain score got all the way down to a 0 or a 1 by the end of the study (this is known as Pain-Free/Nearly Pain-Free), we could consider them cured.

Christie, one of my best therapists, and I traveled to Boulder to provide the treatment. For the next twelve months, we worked with chronic back pain patients. They came from different walks of life and ranged in age from twenty-one to seventy. But they all had one thing in common: chronic back pain that had resisted all medical interventions. Fifty patients were randomly placed in our treatment group, and each received Pain Reprocessing Therapy twice a week for four weeks.

I enjoyed giving Christie pep talks:

Me: We just have to do exactly what we did for Casey. But fifty times in a row. In only eight sessions. And in a different state.

Christie: *Gulp.*

The study was grueling but also really satisfying. We got to know and care for our Boulder patients. We watched as they absorbed the lessons of Pain Reprocessing Therapy and began to break free of the cycle of chronic pain. But would it be enough?

I knew that Pain Reprocessing Therapy works. I had seen it work with my patients in L.A. I had seen it work with Casey. I could see our patients in Boulder improving. But would they improve enough to be cured? Would Pain Reprocessing Therapy hold up under rigorous scientific protocols?

As we reached the end of the study, I was on pins and needles. Finally, Yoni gave me the results. They exceeded even our highest expectations: 98 percent of our patients improved, and 66 percent were Pain-Free/Nearly Pain-Free. Two-thirds of our patients were in the cured category that Yoni didn't even think would be possible. (For the record, Yoni was thrilled with the results.)

The fMRI scans were just as exciting. Dr. Wager and his team didn't just put the patients in the fMRI machine. They put the patients in the fMRI machine and tried to hurt them. The scientists wanted to see how the patients' brains responded to pain, so they used a "back pain evocation device." Which sounds pretty scary, but it turns out it's just an inflatable pillow.

The patient would lie on top of the flat pillow inside the

fMRI machine. Then the scientists would inflate the pillow to put pressure on the patient's back and try to trigger pain. This allowed the researchers to take pictures of the brain while it was feeling pain. Every patient was scanned like this at the beginning of the study and again at the end when they finished treatment.

Once all the scans were done, Yoni toiled over the fMRI data for months. He analyzed millions of data points, corrected for tiny head movements, and compared each patient's before and after scans. Gradually, a pattern emerged: Casey was not a fluke.

Just like Casey, the patients' brains had changed after Pain Reprocessing Therapy. And just like Casey, those changes were centered around the anterior insula—one of Dr. Wager's forty-four pain regions. At the beginning of the study, the pressure from the pillow made the patients' anterior insulas light up like Christmas trees, and they felt a lot of pain. After treatment, their anterior insulas were a lot calmer and the pillow didn't bother them as much. The pillow put the same amount of pressure on their backs in both instances, but after eight sessions of Pain Reprocessing Therapy, their brains responded differently.

Does this mean the anterior insula is the source of chronic pain? Unfortunately, the brain is never that simple. After all, there are forty-three other brain regions involved in pain. But recent research shows that the anterior insula plays an important role in deciding if the brain should generate pain. And incredibly, the patients in our treatment group were able to teach their anterior insulas to make better decisions.

The Boulder Back Pain Study was everything we hoped for.

It validated Pain Reprocessing Therapy, not just as an effective treatment but as the most effective current treatment for chronic pain. By using our system of mind-body techniques, the study patients rewired their brains and turned off their pain. And you can too.

This book will teach you everything you need to know to treat yourself with Pain Reprocessing Therapy. First, I'll explain what neuroplastic pain is and how it develops. Then I'll teach you specific techniques to break the pain cycle and overcome your symptoms. Along the way, there will be plenty of examples, analogies, and patient stories.

To treat your pain, you first need to understand it. So next, we'll explore a fundamental question: What is pain?

CHAPTER 2

Pain Is a Danger Signal

The worst thing about chronic pain is, well, the pain. But the second worst thing is the advice that people give you:

"Try putting ice on it."

"Trying putting heat on it."

"Try stretching."

"Try eating willow bark."

"Try sleeping on a giant magnet."

But the most maddening piece of advice you can get is this:

"Just ignore it."

Some things are impossible to ignore. I learned that my freshman year of college.

I had been up late studying, and I was happily asleep in my dorm room. I was dreaming about acing my econ final when I was jolted awake by the worst sound I had ever heard. Someone had pulled the fire alarm. Now, I'd heard alarms before: smoke alarms, car alarms, sirens. But I had never heard anything like this. It was like a fire truck and a volcano had a baby. A really angry baby that was screaming right in my ear at 4:00 a.m.

I was 100 percent sure that it was just a finals-week prank and that there was no fire. I wanted to ignore it and stay in my warm bed. But ignoring it was not an option. It was just too loud. I got out of bed, went downstairs, and waited outside the building, along with every other student in my dorm. That fire alarm was designed to warn people of danger. And if it could be ignored, it wouldn't be doing its job.

That's what makes the "ignore the pain" advice so unhelpful. Just like that fire alarm, pain is a danger signal. And just like the alarm, pain is designed to be unignorable. Its sole purpose is to let you know that there's a problem. And when your body tells you there's a problem, it makes sure you listen.

Sprain + Brain = Pain!

Imagine you're out on a run. It's a beautiful day. You're enjoying the morning breeze and the sun on your face as you jog with the speed and grace of a gazelle. Your headphones are blasting Bruce Springsteen's greatest hits. Life is good. Until you trip over a tree root and come down awkwardly on your left foot. You feel a sharp twinge in your ankle. It's sprained.

As awful as it feels, that pain is meant to help you. It's your brain's way of saying, "You're at risk of causing further damage to your ankle, so kindly back off until it heals." Without pain, you'd have no idea that you sprained your ankle, you'd keep running, and you'd injure yourself even worse.

Pain doesn't feel good, but it's important. When it works properly, it helps protect our bodies from harm. And as I mentioned in chapter 1, even though pain feels simple, it's actually quite complex. Let's take a closer look at what happened on your morning run:

Breeze is blowing, sun is shining, Springsteen is rocking, etc., etc. . . . *Bam*—you trip.

The instant your foot hits the ground, receptors in your ankle sense the impact and send a signal to your spinal cord. No pain yet.

The signal travels up your spinal cord and into your brain. No pain yet.

The forty-four "pain signature" parts of your brain work together to process the signal and generate the feeling of pain. Now it hurts!

You stop jogging immediately and hobble over to a park bench. You inspect your ankle while Bruce ironically sings "Born to Run."

As you can see, pain was your brain's response to danger signals sent from your ankle. Pain is like a conversation between body and brain. But as in any conversation, sometimes there are misunderstandings.

The Taunt Heard 'Round the World

In 1956, the Cold War was well under way, and the relationship between the United States and the Soviet Union was tense. And at a reception at the Polish embassy in Moscow, it was about to get so much worse. At the event, Soviet premier Nikita Khrushchev gave a speech to Western diplomats. He ended his remarks with a sentence so inflammatory that representatives from thirteen different countries immediately walked out. Khrushchev's final comment was just four simple words, but the next day, it was front-page news all over the world. What was the sentence that inspired so much fear?

"We will bury you!"

Americans were terrified that the leader of a nuclear superpower wanted to destroy them. Tension between the two nations escalated to new heights. "We will bury you!" was a direct threat, and America heard it loud and clear. There was just one problem: Khrushchev never said it. Modern translators believe that Khrushchev's sentence was misinterpreted and that its actual meaning was "We will outlast you!"

That's a big difference. Instead of a threat of nuclear annihilation, it sounds like an expression of confidence. One is terrifying. The other is just a little cocky. A subtle mistranslation changed an innocent boast into a danger signal of nuclear proportions.

Much like Khrushchev's translator, our brains aren't perfect. And sometimes they misinterpret signals from the body. Neuroplastic pain is the result of this type of misunderstanding. It's caused by your brain misinterpreting normal messages from your body as if they were dangerous. The body is fine, but the brain creates pain anyway. In other words, neuroplastic pain is a false alarm.

Brain Mistakes and Sudden Aches

In 1995, the *British Medical Journal* reported on the case of a construction worker who accidentally jumped down onto a six-inch nail. Yikes! The nail went all the way through his boot and out the other side. He was in agony.

His coworkers rushed him to the emergency room, and doctors carefully extracted the nail. When they took off his boot to assess the damage, they were stunned to discover no blood, no puncture wound, not even a scratch. By some miracle, the nail had gone right in between his toes!

Why did he feel pain? He saw a nail go through his boot and assumed that he was injured. This changed the way his brain processed signals from his body. His foot was just sending normal signals—the texture of his sock, the tightness of his boot, the unfamiliar feeling of a nail between his toes. These are harmless sensations, but his brain was expecting danger signals, so it processed them as pain, pain, pain.

What happened to the construction worker was a freak accident, but scientists can actually replicate this experience. Researchers at a medical school in Texas recruited people for a study. They wanted to see if they could trick the brain into feeling pain. The subjects were hooked up to a machine with electrodes placed on their heads. The scientists told the participants that the machine was going to send an electrical current through their heads and cause a temporary headache. But it was all a ruse. The machine didn't actually do anything. To really sell it, the machine had a big sign on it that said SHOCK GENERATOR. (Texans aren't known for their subtlety.)

The scientists turned on the machine. A nearby speaker made a humming sound so that it seemed like the machine was doing something. The participants thought that electricity was going through their heads. And guess what? They felt pain. Just like in the case of the construction worker, their brains made a mistake. Their bodies were just sending normal, safe signals, but their brains processed them as pain. Why does the brain misinterpret signals like this? I'll answer that in chapter 3.

For now, the important point is that the pain-processing parts of the brain aren't perfect. Sometimes they make mistakes. Of course, making a mistake every once in a while isn't a big deal. The real problem is when the brain makes a mistake and it sticks.

Our Changing Brains

The blue wildebeest is a large antelope with curved horns that lives in Africa. The wildebeests aren't exactly blue; they're more of a bluish gray. Adult blue wildebeests are pretty normal: they graze, they migrate, they try not to get eaten by predators. Blue wildebeest babies, on the other hand, are amazing.

Wildebeest calves are born in the middle of the herd to keep them safe, but they don't need protecting for long. Baby wildebeests can stand on their own an average of six minutes after birth. Within thirty minutes of being born, they can walk. And within a day of birth, they can outrun a hyena! Now, hyenas can run 30 to 35 miles per hour, so that's quite a feat. By way of comparison, Usain Bolt, who has eight Olympic gold medals for sprinting, has been clocked at a maximum speed of 27.44 miles per hour. Which means that a one-day-old baby wildebeest is faster than the fastest man alive.

Baby humans, on the other hand, are less impressive. They are certainly cute and chubby, but at birth a baby can do almost nothing. Twenty-four hours later, a baby can do . . . still nothing. Don't get me wrong. Some of my best friends are humans, but let's be honest: we are born with no skills.

That's okay, though, because we are born with something even better: big, beautiful brains that excel at learning new abilities. It takes months instead of minutes, but we do learn to stand up. We can't do it when we're half an hour old, but we do start walking and eventually running. We may never run faster than blue wildebeests, but we surpass them in other ways. We learn to read and write, drive cars, and adjust our alarm clocks after daylight saving time. We don't succeed at any of those things the first time we try them, but we master them through practice.

Human brains are amazing because of how much they can learn and change and develop. It sounds magical, but it's just basic biology. The brain is a collection of neurons (nerve cells) that talk to one another. How do neurons talk? By firing short electrical bursts. And the more they talk to one another, the better they get at it.

Think of a baby trying to walk for the first time. His young brain has no idea what to do. Neurons in his brain fire and trigger other neurons, but because it's the first time, the pattern is unfamiliar and clumsy. He falls. But he's determined and he tries again. This time the connections between his adorable little neurons are a tiny bit stronger. He's just slightly more stable. The more he practices, the better these particular neurons get at working together. Eventually, his brain learns: push off, lean slightly forward, keep your balance, step, and repeat. With enough repetition, it'll become automatic, and he won't even need to think about it.

As scientists like to say, "Neurons that fire together, wire together." Once these patterns of neurons (or "neural pathways") are wired together, complex tasks feel easy: tying a shoelace, playing the guitar, taking a really good selfie that looks like you aren't trying too hard.

Learning Pain

Our brains are great at learning useful skills, but the dark side is that they are also great at learning bad habits. Like pain. When the brain experiences pain over and over, those neurons get "wired together," and they get better and better at firing together. Unfortunately, that means the brain gets better and better at feeling pain. If a brain gets too good at experiencing pain, the condition can become chronic. Basically, your brain can unintentionally learn how to be in pain.

That's the origin of the term "neuroplastic pain." "Neuro" refers to the brain and other parts of the nervous system; "plastic" means developed or changed. Neuroplastic pain is when the brain changes in such a way that reinforces chronic pain.

One of the most important pain studies of the last few years actually captured this process in action. Researchers followed people who had recently injured their backs. At first, their pain was active in the normal pain regions of the brain. But when the pain became chronic, it shifted to parts of the brain associated with learning and memory.

Neuroplastic pain is a fundamentally different kind of pain. It's pain that has gotten stuck because your brain has learned it too well. The good news is that just as your brain can learn pain, it can unlearn it. Pain Reprocessing Therapy retrains your brain to interpret signals from your body properly. Over time, this rewires your brain and deactivates your pain.

Plain Pain or Brain Pain?

Now that you know the difference between normal pain and neuroplastic pain, it raises the question: If you're in pain, how do you know which one you have? I've done many intakes with pain patients, and one of the first things I do is assess whether their symptoms are likely to be neuroplastic or caused by structural problems in the body.

These are some of the questions I ask:

- Have medical treatments been ineffective or just given you temporary relief?
- Did the pain come on during a stressful time in your life?
- Do you have (or have you had) symptoms in multiple parts of your body?
- Is your pain inconsistent in terms of where and when it appears and how severe it is?
- Do you think about the pain often or all the time? Does it worry you throughout the day?

I wish this were like a magazine quiz and I could give you five points for every "yes" answer. But it's not that simple. There is no definitive checklist. While "yes" answers are associated with neuroplastic pain, we assess everyone on a case-by-case basis.

As I said in chapter 1, neuroplastic chronic pain is more common than structurally caused chronic pain.

How much more common?

In the Boulder Back Pain Study, there were fifty subjects in the treatment group. Dr. Howard Schubiner, who specializes in pain, did a medical consultation, and I did a more general evaluation. Based on our initial assessments, as well as evidence we gathered during treatment, we found no cases of chronic back pain that we believed to be structurally caused. None!

You may be thinking, "Of course you thought everyone had neuroplastic pain. You specialize in neuroplastic pain. When all you have is a hammer, everything looks like a nail." Well, my hypothetically skeptical friend, that couldn't be further from the truth. We went into the study expecting some of the patients to have structurally induced pain. But to our surprise, we didn't find evidence of a single case. Even patients who had significant findings on X-rays or MRIs ended up having neuroplastic pain. We know this because Pain Reprocessing Therapy successfully eliminated their pain.

One of the patients had scoliosis at a seventy-three-degree angle. Essentially, her spine looked like the letter *S*. Yet by the end of the study, she overcame all her symptoms.

Another patient was a former college linebacker. He'd spent years pounding into offensive linemen at full speed. As a result of his time playing football, he had two large disc herniations with partial nerve-root compression. He hadn't been able to sit, stand, or walk without pain for thirty years.

Despite these physical findings, he was pain-free by the end of treatment.

The Boulder study focused on back pain, but it mirrors my experiences treating people with every form of pain. In most cases, pain caused by a physical problem will not become chronic. It will heal or respond to medical treatment. Most chronic pain is neuroplastic pain.

However, I am by no means an absolutist. Some patients *do* have structurally caused chronic pain. You never want to assume that your pain is neuroplastic without sufficient evidence. It's important to be thorough. I've included an appendix in the back of the book—it's a guide to help you determine whether your pain is neuroplastic or caused by a physical problem in your body.

Bottom Line: Pain Is Good, Neuroplastic Pain Is Bad

Normally, pain is helpful. It doesn't feel good, but it's an important danger signal that helps protect our bodies. Neuroplastic pain, on the other hand, is a mistake. Neuroplastic pain is caused by the brain misinterpreting safe signals from the body as if they were dangerous. So, we feel pain even when there is no damage to the body.

Because our brains are good at learning, neuroplastic pain can get stuck. Pain leads to neurons getting wired together, which leads to more pain.

To get rid of neuroplastic pain, we need to look at the reason the brain misinterprets safe signals in the first place. Once we understand why the brain makes this critical mistake, we can focus on preventing it. Then we can harness the brain's amazing flexibility to develop new neural pathways. Using Pain Reprocessing Therapy, we can rewire the brain and unlearn painful symptoms.

So, what is the root cause of neuroplastic pain?

Why do our brains make this mistake?

What is the fuel that keeps the pain going?

Fear.

CHAPTER 3

Nothing to Fear but Fear Itself

"What if I'm the *one* person who can't get better?"

I was sitting in my office with Joe, a new patient with chronic neck pain. I could see how anxious he was.*

"I'm confident you can recover," I said. "You're a great candidate for treatment."

"What if I do get better," he said, worried, "and then the pain comes back?"

Joe's mind was churning out one scary thought after another.

"If that happens, you'll get better again," I said. "You're very motivated."

His eyes suddenly widened. "What if I'm *too* motivated?"

Joe was feeling fear.

---

* All patients in this book have given permission for their cases to be presented. I've changed their names to protect their privacy.

Throughout history, many great thinkers have contemplated the nature of fear. Gandhi said that fear was our enemy. Mandela felt that it was a challenge to overcome. Yoda said that it was "the path to the dark side."

But at its core, fear is simple. It's what we feel when we think we're in danger. Fear is universal, and we all experience it daily:

That feeling you get when you see a police car in your rearview mirror? Fear.

That feeling you get when you accidentally like your ex's Instagram post? Fear.

That feeling you get when your cell phone slips out of your hand and into the toilet? Fear. (And a little relief because you spend way too much time on Instagram and maybe it was a blessing in disguise.)

Fear puts us in a state of high alert. It's the brain's way of saying, "Danger! Danger! Danger!"

Lions and Zebras and Fears, Oh My!

Imagine two zebras: Nervous Nick and Fearless Frank. As you might guess from his name, Nervous Nick has a lot of fear. He's always afraid. Always on high alert. Constantly scanning the savanna for threats. His motto is "Did you guys hear that?!"

Fearless Frank, on the other hand, is trotting around like he owns the place. He's downright relaxed. He's nibbling on some grass without a care in the world. Maybe he'll take a nap later.

At first glance, Fearless Frank seems like he has it all figured out. He's like that cool kid in high school who never seemed worried about anything. Except that cool kid didn't get ambushed by lions and eaten on the way to his locker. But that's exactly what just happened to Frank. Without fear to protect him, Frank didn't see the lions until it was too late.

What about Nervous Nick? Five minutes ago, he noticed a slight rustling in the bushes, and he immediately made a run for it. Because he was on high alert, Nick lived to be nervous another day.

Nick's fear made him more sensitive to danger, so he spotted a subtle threat. That's fear's job. And it's just as true for humans as it is for zebras. Fear helps us identify danger, so it magnifies potential threats in order to protect us. Noises seem louder when we're afraid. And people are more sensitive to smell when they're on high alert.

But fear doesn't just magnify our senses. Fear also amplifies danger signals like pain.

A group of researchers proved this using terrifying pictures and a hot probe. Fun! In this experiment, people got hot pulses on their skin randomly while looking through a series of photos. Some of the pictures were scary, while others were neutral. Even though the pulses were all the same, the subjects experienced much more pain when looking at the scary photos.

What's really interesting is that sometimes the participants felt pain when there was no hot pulse at all. But this happened only when they were looking at the scary photos, not the neutral ones. The fear from the pictures put their brains on high alert, and they experienced pain even when the probe was off.

This is the key to understanding neuroplastic pain. Being in a state of high alert can change the way we perceive signals from our body. Fear can create pain.

In this chapter, I'm going to explain the origins of fear and why some of us have a tendency to be on high alert. Then I'm going to present three case studies showing how fear can turn into pain. Finally, I'll teach you how fear keeps neuroplastic pain stuck in a loop and tell you what we're going to do about it.

Getting to the Source

Constantly being on high alert is a great strategy if you're trying to avoid lions in the Serengeti. But for many of us living in the modern world, excess fear is a burden that makes our lives harder and our pain worse. Where does all this fear come from?

There are many different factors that can put us in a state of high alert.

Some of the patients I've worked with were in very stressful situations when their pain first appeared. They may have just started a high-pressure job or recently ended a long-term relationship. Even joyous occasions can put us in a state of high alert. I've had patients develop pain weeks before a wedding, and others whose pain began after getting a promotion. Big life changes, both positive and negative, can generate feelings of stress and put our brains on high alert.

With other patients, it's less about current stressors and more about the past. Some people experience events in their childhood that make them prone to fear—things like having a troubled family dynamic, struggling in school, or being bullied. This type of early adversity can lead to general feelings of being unsafe that last far beyond childhood. Studies show that people who have experienced early-life stress are more sensitive to fear.

Finally, certain behaviors can bring us to a state of high alert without our even realizing it. There are three habits I see again and again in my patients that trigger fear and aggravate neuroplastic pain: worrying, putting pressure on yourself, and self-criticism. Here's a breakdown of how each of these can lead to a state of high alert:

WORRYING

"Supposing a tree fell down, Pooh, when we were underneath it?" asked Piglet.

"Supposing it didn't," said Pooh.

Much like Piglet, many of us worry about things that could happen, things that might happen, things that have already happened.

"Is my boss mad at me?"

"Am I going to get enough sleep?"

"Is there spinach stuck in my teeth?"

Regardless of whether these worries are about your job, your schedule, or your dental hygiene, they can increase feelings of danger and put your brain on high alert.

PUTTING PRESSURE ON YOURSELF

When I point out to patients that they put a lot of pressure on themselves, they often respond, "You're right. I *have* to stop doing that immediately!" But not surprisingly, pressuring ourselves to stop pressuring ourselves isn't the best strategy.

We live in a culture that places a strong emphasis on perfection, so it's no surprise that many of us put pressure on ourselves.

"I have to get an A on my test!"

"I need to lose five pounds before my wedding!"

"I must meditate for twenty minutes a day!"

These thoughts may seem innocent, but pressure triggers parts of the brain associated with fear and vigilance. Pressure puts us on high alert and keeps us in a state of fear.

SELF-CRITICISM

Claude Monet is one of the most famous painters of all time. He was the father of Impressionism, and his paintings sold for enormous sums. Yet despite his talent and success, Monet was intensely self-critical.

Here are some statements that he made about himself:

"I'm not a great painter."

"I'm making stupid mistakes."

"What I'm doing is just dreadful."

"My life has been nothing but a failure and all that's left for me to do is to destroy my paintings before I disappear."

Yikes!

It's no surprise that the French prime minister called Monet "the king of the grumps." (It sounds even better in French: *le roi des grincheux*.)

Much like Monet, many chronic pain patients are very hard on themselves. They ignore their achievements and beat themselves up for minor mistakes. But self-criticism doesn't just make you a *grincheux*; it also puts your brain on high alert. Neuroscientists have shown that criticism activates the brain's threat system, so it's another trigger for fear.

The Way In

High levels of fear set the stage for neuroplastic pain. But the pain itself can start in different ways.

Neuroplastic pain can start with an injury or appear out of nowhere. The onset can be sudden or gradual. The pain can appear during a stressful time or when nothing particularly difficult is going on.

To demonstrate this, let's look at three patients who developed pain in three different ways:

GRADUAL ONSET

Melanie grew up with a fearful mom and an anxious dad. As a result of her upbringing, she worried constantly.

If she went on a bad first date, she'd think, "What if I never meet anyone and I end up alone?"

If she went on a good first date, she'd think, "What if we fall in love and he cheats on me?"

After living in a state of fear for twenty-seven years, Melanie started getting tension headaches. At first, they appeared only a couple of times a week, but after a few months, they became chronic.

She stopped going out socially. It took too much energy to pretend that she was okay.

For ten months, she stayed at home, depressed that she was missing out on life, worried that her pain would never go away.

STRESSFUL SITUATION

Leah was a violin prodigy. She was accepted to one of the best college music programs in the country when she was only sixteen. But living away from home, and sharing a dorm with students several years older than she was, Leah found herself feeling overwhelmed. By the end of the first month, she had arm and wrist pain so severe that she could barely lift her bow. The stress of being in a new environment with so much pressure put her in a state of high alert and triggered neuroplastic pain.

Concerned about aggravating her symptoms, Leah didn't play the violin again for seven years.

INITIAL INJURY

James had an extremely demanding job with long hours and endless responsibilities. He got new emails faster than he could read them. James blew off steam on the weekends by playing basketball. But one day he was out on the court and suffered a bad back sprain—walking hurt, sitting hurt, pretty much everything except standing hurt.

After a week or two, his muscle strain healed, but his pain persisted.

James became fixated on his back pain. He started using heating pads and back pillows at work, frequently checking his body to see if the pain was better or worse. Eventually, he had to buy a standing desk just to get through the day.

To Fear or Not to Fear

To give you a little closure, these stories all have happy endings. All three patients are now pain-free. Melanie is socializing with her friends again. Leah is teaching music. And James is back at his old desk. (Though he's still behind on his emails.)

Melanie, Leah, and James developed their pain through different routes. But they have two important things in common. First, their pain arose in an environment of fear. And second, once their pain appeared, they all responded the same way: with fear of the pain itself. Melanie was worried that her pain was permanent. Leah was anxious about making her symptoms worse. James was preoccupied with his back. These are all forms of fear. And fear of the pain itself is what keeps neuroplastic pain alive.

As I explained in chapter 2, neuroplastic pain is a mistake.

It's your brain misinterpreting safe signals from your body as if they were dangerous. It's a false alarm. And the way you react to that false alarm makes all the difference. If you respond with fear, it reinforces the pain. In this way, pain is like an impressionable toddler.

Safety vs. Danger

My two-year-old niece is incredibly rambunctious. The day she learned how to walk, she learned how to run, and ever since then, she runs everywhere.

But her ambition exceeds her coordination, and she falls down a lot. There's a moment just after she falls when she looks at you and waits to see how you'll react before deciding how she feels. If you run over to her, concerned, worried, frantically asking if she's okay, she'll start crying, convinced that she must have taken quite a spill. If instead, you calmly say, "Hey, it looks like you took a little stumble," she's back up and running before you even finish your sentence.

The way you react reinforces either a sense of danger or a sense of safety. And it works the same way with neuroplastic pain.

Pain is a danger signal. And in the case of neuroplastic pain, the way we react determines whether this signal stays on or switches off. When we respond to the pain with fear, it reinforces that it's dangerous, and the pain persists.

Fear is the fuel for the pain.

A study in the Netherlands showed this phenomenon in action. The researchers recruited people with low back pain and measured how much pain-related fear they had. When they followed up six months later, the people who scored high on fear were much more likely to still be in pain. This was true regardless of how bad their pain was initially or how long they'd had it.

The Dutch scientists looked at back pain, but dozens of studies on everything from headaches to knee pain to fibromyalgia all show the same pattern. The more fear you have around your pain, the more likely your pain is to continue.

And this can lead to an unfortunate loop.

Stuck in a Feedback Loop

Nothing is better than an amazing first date. You're sitting across from this person you just met, but it's as if you've known each other for years. You're finishing each other's sentences and getting lost in each other's eyes. By dessert, you guys are picking out baby names.

My friend Chris recently went on a date with a girl named Molly and . . . it was the exact opposite of that. Chris and Molly met online, and they'd been texting each other for a couple of weeks. Over text, everything was great: jokes, banter, emojis, they had it all.

When they finally met for their first date, Chris had very high expectations. He really wanted to make a good impression, but he was super nervous. And soon, a terrible cycle developed.

It started innocently enough. Chris made a joke, and Molly didn't laugh. Which made him feel a little more anxious. So he told a story that went on for way too long. Molly started fidgeting and looking at her watch. Then Chris really started to freak out. His panic clouded his judgment, and he committed the worst first-date sin of all: he launched into the epic tale of his last breakup. Soon Molly was looking around like a *Titanic* passenger searching for a lifeboat.

The more nervous Chris got, the worse Molly felt; the worse Molly felt, the more nervous Chris got. The cycle continued until the waiter mercifully brought the check.

This is called a feedback loop, in which a behavior and the response to that behavior can create a never-ending cycle. Pain and fear can get locked in a similar feedback loop, which causes neuroplastic pain to become chronic. Here's how it happens:

1. Pain triggers feelings of fear.
2. The fear puts the brain on high alert, which causes more pain.
3. Which leads to more fear.
4. Which leads to more pain.

The more afraid you are of the pain, the more likely your pain is to get stuck and stay stuck. It's a downward spiral that we call the pain-fear cycle.

Me and My Knee (and Fear Makes Three)

Long before I learned about the pain-fear cycle, I was living in the pain-fear cycle. One of my biggest struggles was with pain in my left knee. The pain started off small, but having dealt with chronic back pain, I had a lot of fear. I was immediately consumed by fear thoughts: "What if the pain doesn't go away? What if my knee gets worse? What if I can't go dancing?" (I hate dancing, but fear thoughts are not very rational.)

I started treating my knee as if it were made of glass. I kept my leg elevated whenever I sat down. I was careful to never put too much weight on that side. I was constantly thinking about my knee, obsessing about my knee, scanning it for the slightest twinge. I was on full high alert.

The more I focused on my knee, the more fear I felt. And the more fear I felt, the more I focused on my knee. Surprise, surprise, my knee stayed in pain.

My fear of chronic pain turned my pain chronic.

Fear by Another Name

Many of my patients immediately relate to the concept of fear. They feel scared of their pain, and they're eager to explore that dynamic. I've had other patients who didn't identify with the word "fear." Not because they didn't have fear, but because they called it something else.

One patient said it wasn't really fear that she felt around her pain but frustration. Another patient said he mostly felt despair. These feelings may seem like they're different from fear, but they fall under the same umbrella.

When I discuss emotions with my patients, I ask a simple question: "Does this feeling make your brain feel more danger or less danger?" If the answer is "more danger," then it's a form of fear. So when I talk about fear of the pain, I'm including frustration, despair, stress, anguish, anxiety, annoyance, dismay, and anything else that puts you on high alert.

Patient Perspective

The pain started on my fortieth birthday. It was a big milestone, and I wasn't where I thought I would be in life. I was divorced and single, my kids were getting older, and I had an underlying fear that I would be alone for the rest of my life.

Of course, at the time, I didn't realize that turning forty was what did it. I thought my back hurt because I had gardened too much the day before. Over the next few years I tried everything: I saw a chiropractor. I tried a physical therapist. Tried yoga. Tried a different kind of yoga hoping it would get deeper into my muscles. Then I kind of gave up and said, "This is just part of me now."

Being in pain was depressing. My whole mindset changed. Before the pain started, I was a positive, optimistic, outgoing, love-to-have-fun person. But after, it was hard to even smile sometimes. Everything was a gray fog.

I have a pretty high threshold for pain. There's not a whole lot that scares me. I wouldn't say I was fearful of the pain. It was more like I felt beat down. I tried all these different things, but it was like brick wall after brick wall, dead end after dead end. I just felt defeated.

When I learned about neuroplastic pain, I started seeing the pain in a new way. At first I was hopeless, because I didn't think it was going to change. But eventually, when I had the tools, I realized I was in control and it doesn't have to be that way. I went from feeling like I was at the pain's mercy to feeling like I had the power back.

—LINDSAY

Breaking the Pain-Fear Cycle

To recap, when you have neuroplastic pain, the fear you feel around the pain reinforces that it's dangerous, and the pain persists. Which leads to more fear. Which leads to more pain. And the cycle continues.

Whether you've been in pain for months, years, or decades, there's a simple and straightforward way to break this cycle. We need to eliminate your fear. We need to teach your brain that the pain is not dangerous. This is the first goal of Pain Reprocessing Therapy. "Reprocessing" means changing the way your brain interprets the pain.

Of course, overcoming the fear of your pain is easier said than done. Pain is inherently scary. It's hard not to be afraid of something that hurts! But when you can respond to your pain without fear, you'll calm your brain, expose the false alarm, and deactivate your pain.

In chapters 4 through 6, I'll teach you proven techniques to turn off your danger signals and break out of the pain-fear cycle. But that's just the beginning. We don't just want to change your relationship with fear around your pain. We want to change your relationship with all fear.

Potatoes, Pumpkin Pie, and Pain

Every Thanksgiving, I can count on three things: loads of turkey, tons of football, and a half dozen of my patients calling me because their pain has flared up. Spending time with family is great, but it can also cause a lot of stress. Your cousins are drinking too much, your siblings are arguing about politics, your mom's asking you to show her how to print out an email attachment. Again.

It's a lot to handle, and it can put you in a state of high alert, which magnifies danger signals and makes your pain worse. Just as we're going to target the fear around your pain, we're going to address these more general types of fear and stress. This is the second goal of Pain Reprocessing Therapy: to foster an overall sense of safety. By "turning down the volume knob" on danger, we can neutralize neuroplastic pain at the root. In chapters 7 through 9, I'll teach you specific strategies to help you go from high alert to low alert. Even on Thanksgiving.

What's Next?

Most likely, if you're reading this, you're in pain. And you've realized that the old ways of doing things are not working. I'm here to offer you a new way. I've described the neuroscience of pain. I've explained how it can become chronic. I've told you that fear is the fuel for neuroplastic pain. Now it's time to do something about it.

You have all the background information you need. The rest of this book is about healing your pain. I'm going to give you the tools you need to break out of the pain-fear cycle. I'm going to teach you how to use them and when to use them.

As a former chronic pain sufferer, I know the struggle. I know you've probably gone through a lot to get here. But I want you to have hope. I know the power of Pain Reprocessing Therapy. It's been validated by a rigorous scientific study. It's helped my patients. It helped me. And if you have neuroplastic pain, I know it will help you too.

Let's begin.

CHAPTER 4

Embracing a New Perspective

It was 9:00 p.m., California time, which meant it was midnight in Michigan. I glanced at my phone. I thought about waiting until the morning, but I was feeling desperate. I couldn't wait. So I started to dial.

By December 2008, I'd been out of pain for a couple of years. Life was good again . . . until the night of the accident. I had a great day leading up to it—I got lunch with a friend, worked out at the gym, and went to see that movie where Brad Pitt ages backward (spoiler alert: he dies of old age as a baby).

As I was waiting to exit the movie theater parking lot, I saw that a car was headed straight toward me. I blasted my horn, but it was too late. He crashed into my passenger-side door.

The driver was very apologetic and assured me that his insurance company would fix my car. There was just one small problem: my back was in agony.

By the time I got home, I was close to panic:

"Did the accident mess up my spine?"

"Or is this just my neuroplastic pain rearing its ugly head?"

It was late at night, I was in pain, and I was terrified. So I did what any reasonable person would do. I called one of the world's leading experts on diagnosing pain.

You might remember Dr. Howard Schubiner from earlier in the book. He evaluated the patients in the Boulder Back Pain Study to determine whether their pain was neuroplastic or caused by structural problems. Dr. Schubiner is a board-certified internist and the founder of the Mind Body Medicine Program at Providence Hospital in Michigan. He's brilliant and insightful, but best of all, he doesn't turn off his ringer when he goes to sleep.

Dr. Schubiner (*groggy*): Hello?

Me: Howard, I need your help! A car crashed into my passenger-side door, and now my back's killing me. I'm not sure if it's neuroplastic or structural.

Dr. Schubiner (*alarmed*): How fast was the other car going?

Me: Five miles per hour.

(*Dr. Schubiner laughs.*)

Me: You don't think it was fast enough to cause structural damage to my back?

Dr. Schubiner: Alan, I don't think it was fast enough to move the water molecules in your body.

To this day, I have no idea what water molecules had to do with anything, but I felt reassured. My brain calmed down, and over the next couple of hours, my back pain dissipated completely.

The Moral of the Story

What can we learn from my car accident, besides the fact that Howard Schubiner is a really nice guy? After the accident, I developed pain . . . which led to fear, which led to more pain. I had fallen right back into the pain-fear cycle.

But I didn't just have fear of the pain. I had a very specific fear—that the pain was caused by a physical problem in my back. I was scared of the pain because I thought it meant that something was broken, or ruptured, or otherwise damaged in my body.

And this is the exact fear that fuels neuroplastic pain. When we're in pain, we naturally conclude that there's a physical cause.

Maybe we believe it's inflammation or scar tissue or arthritis. Maybe we think it's a disc problem, or a nerve issue, or a curved spine. Maybe we suspect it's poor posture or muscle weakness or a vitamin deficiency. Regardless of the specifics, at a core level, all chronic pain patients have the same fear: "There has to be *something* going on in my body that's causing this."

And when the brain believes that the body is damaged, it responds with pain.

But when you can embrace a different belief—that the pain is due to your brain making a mistake and that your body is fine—then the fear goes away. And soon after, the pain fades.

Which brings us back to my car accident. Once Dr. Schubiner explained that the collision couldn't have caused a physical problem in my back, the fear went away. I still felt pain for a little bit, but I was able to look at it differently. I knew it was a false alarm.

By eliminating fear, I had taken away the fuel for the pain. Within a few hours, my brain stopped interpreting the pain as dangerous, and the pain disappeared.

To eliminate neuroplastic pain, we need to accept that there's no physical problem in the body. It's possible. I've done it, and I've helped my patients do it. But it's not easy. And there are three main barriers to overcome.

BARRIER 1: BIOLOGY

Many of my patients have a hard time believing that their pain could be caused by their brains. Even if they believe it logically, on a gut level they feel like there *has* to be something wrong with their bodies.

There's a simple reason for this: biology. Over millions of years of evolution, we've been wired to link physical pain with physical injury in order to protect ourselves.

What would happen if we didn't have this biological instinct? Well, just ask Pete Reiser.

Pete Reiser was one of the best baseball players of all time, but there's a reason that you've never heard of him. His career ended before it really began. Pete had everything you could want in a baseball player—power, speed, a really cool nickname (Pistol Pete) . . . But one thing he didn't have was common sense.

Whenever Pete would get injured, he'd just keep playing. He broke his arm and kept throwing for weeks. He fractured his ankle and batted the next day. No matter how bad the injury, Pete refused to let his body heal, and his playing career was eventually cut short.

We've been wired to link pain with physical injury to prevent this exact problem. When we get injured, we know to give our bodies time to heal, and soon after, we're good as new.

But in the case of neuroplastic pain, this biological instinct holds us back from recovery. Our brains are telling us, "There's something wrong with your body!" Even though there isn't.

To overcome this barrier, we need to embrace a perspective that's counterintuitive: "My pain makes me feel like I have a physical injury, but in this case, it's actually a false alarm."

BARRIER 2: CONDITIONED RESPONSES

In the late 1960s, comedian Steve Martin was on top of the world. His career was taking off, he was making good money, and he was dating up a storm. But then one night, it all came crashing down. He was out with his friends when, out of nowhere, he had a crippling panic attack.

"My heart began to race above two hundred beats per minute," he said. "The saliva drained from my mouth so completely that I could not move my tongue."

The next day he was feeling better, but that evening, he had another panic attack.

His brain had developed an unfortunate connection: He came to associate nighttime with anxiety. And this association lasted for months. During the day he was fine, but as soon as the sun set, he was a mess. This is called a conditioned response—his brain connected a physical symptom with a neutral trigger.

Evolutionarily speaking, conditioned responses are helpful. If you eat a poisonous berry and get sick, your brain creates an association. It puts a DANGER sign up, and after that, just the smell of that berry can make you nauseated. Conditioned responses can protect us from repeating dangerous behaviors.

But what if that berry wasn't poisonous? What if you just happened to catch a stomach bug shortly after eating it? Your brain—not taking any chances—might create an association anyway, and put a DANGER sign up on food that's actually safe.

This type of conditioned response is very common in people with neuroplastic pain. It happens when pain becomes linked with a physical position or activity. The pain isn't caused by the position or activity; rather, the brain creates an association between the two. And this association can make us think that there's something structurally wrong with our bodies.

During my chronic pain days, I developed a number of conditioned responses. When I had knee pain, walking was the trigger. When I had shoulder pain, it hurt just to put on a jacket. When I had neck pain, I couldn't turn my head to the left (which made changing lanes on the freeway particularly tricky).

But the worst conditioned response of all was sitting. Within minutes of sitting down, my back began to hurt. The longer I sat, the worse it got. And it was specific too. Hard chairs were worse than soft chairs. Short chairs were worse than tall chairs. Don't even get me started on benches.

I became a chair expert. I knew which movie theaters were the most comfortable. I knew which restaurant had the best seats. (Answer: Makai Lounge . . . so tall, so cushy.)

But in truth, the chairs themselves weren't causing my back pain, no matter how much it seemed like they were. My brain had just formed a certain connection (sitting = dangerous). The chairs would trigger pain, not because they put pressure on my spine, but because my brain had developed an association. There was nothing inherently bad about nighttime that caused Steve Martin's anxiety. And there was nothing inherently bad about chairs that caused my pain. We both had very strong conditioned responses.

How do I know it was a conditioned response and not the chairs that were causing my pain? Because now I can sit in any type of chair for any length of time with no pain. My back hasn't changed. The chairs haven't changed. The only thing that's changed is that I unlearned the conditioned response.

Conditioned responses can make it hard to believe that your pain is caused by your brain. If you have back pain every time you sit, it makes sense to think it's the sitting that's causing your pain. After all, everything you've ever learned about cause and effect is telling you that's what it is.

But if you have neuroplastic pain, it isn't the sitting, or standing, or walking that's causing your pain. It's a conditioned response. Your brain has developed an association between a position or activity and the onset of pain. But just as these associations can be learned, they can be unlearned.

BARRIER 3: MEDICAL DIAGNOSES

Modern medicine is rooted in something called the biomedical model, which focuses on treating a condition by finding a single, structural cause and fixing it.

When you suffer an injury, the biomedical model can be really helpful. For example, imagine you injure your wrist trying to slam dunk on a children's basketball hoop (don't laugh—it could happen to anyone). First, a physician will take an X-ray to make sure there's no fracture. Then they'll examine you to determine the degree of the sprain. Finally, they'll give you a brace to immobilize your wrist for a few weeks, allowing it to heal. Score one for modern medicine.

But in the case of chronic pain, the biomedical model often

hurts more than it helps. Doctors are trained to look for structural causes. And when you look for structural issues, you're likely to find some, even if they aren't actually causing the problem.

Many chronic pain sufferers have been given diagnoses by physicians: degenerative disc disease, repetitive-strain injury, fibromyalgia, the list goes on and on.

Sometimes these diagnoses are actually comforting. Having pain and not knowing why is terrible. The uncertainty can be overwhelming. When you're given an explanation for your symptoms, it can bring enormous relief. But there's a downside to these medical diagnoses. They reinforce the idea that there's something wrong with your body, even if there isn't.

I mentioned this in chapter 2, but it's worth repeating: most chronic pain is neuroplastic. We may develop wear and tear, we may suffer injuries, but our bodies are quite robust and resilient.

Patient Perspective

I had all kinds of pain. I had pain in my knees, feet, rib cage, and shoulder. But the pain that kept me up at night was my wrist pain. I bounced around from doctor to doctor, trying to find out what was wrong with my wrists. Most of them told me it was tendonitis.

The internet was my worst enemy. I would go on tendonitis websites, and they'd say that you have to ice your wrists for TWO HOURS a day, and if you keep using them, you'll deteriorate your tendons further. I was so worried that they were going to get worse and worse.

I couldn't think about anything else. So I couldn't talk about anything else. I couldn't connect with my friends anymore. It was incredibly isolating. My life had just stopped. I needed to devote all my attention and energy to getting better. It felt like quicksand.

When I learned that my brain could be causing my pain, I thought, "This makes so much sense and I'm so inspired." But there was also a part of me saying, "BUT WHAT IF THIS IS ALL WRONG, AND IT'S GOING TO GET SO MUCH WORSE?"

It was hard to let go of these structural beliefs because I'd been reinforcing them for three or four years. It took a couple months of uncertainty and going back and forth before I was able to accept that there was nothing wrong with my body.

Once that belief really stuck, it was incredibly liberating. Even before the pain totally went away, I felt freed and powerful. I started going back to school, started driving again, was in classes again . . . I remember sitting in the cafeteria one day and thinking, "I'm out in the world. This is amazing. I'm a person again. I'm a whole person again."

—EMMET

OVERCOMING BARRIERS

These three barriers can make it difficult to accept that our pain is neuroplastic. They reinforce the belief that chronic pain is coming from our bodies, keeping us stuck in the pain-fear cycle.

Luckily, there's a single solution to overcoming these barriers: evidence. The more evidence you have that there's nothing wrong with your body, the easier it is to believe that your brain is the culprit.

And the most compelling type of evidence is when your pain deviates from its normal pattern. I discovered this in a rather unlikely place.

Searching for Exceptions

I had chronic back pain for two long years. During that time, I saw a team of physicians, physical therapists, chiropractors, and acupuncturists. But the team that helped me the most was the Los Angeles Lakers.

In April 2006, I went to a basketball game. Sitting was always painful for me, but I wasn't about to miss my hometown Lakers playing the Phoenix Suns in the playoffs. And what a game! In the fourth quarter, the Lakers made a thrilling comeback and hit a last-second shot to push it into overtime. The crowd went crazy! Overtime was even more exciting, and they made *another* last-second shot to win the game.

It was pandemonium!

But nobody in the stadium was more excited than I was, because for the first time in two years, I was sitting without pain.

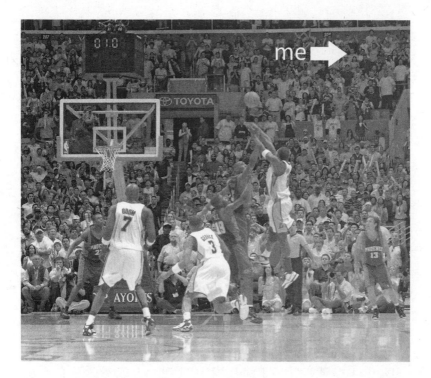

Sometimes when we're enjoying the moment, we deprive our pain of its one fuel source: fear. I was so absorbed in the game that I turned off the danger signals in my brain without even realizing it. In other words, the Lakers distracted me out of the pain-fear cycle!

I had just gotten my first piece of evidence that my pain wasn't caused by sitting. How could it be? I'd been sitting for three hours, and my back was feeling fine!

This is called an exception—an instance when the pain behaves differently from how it would if it were actually caused by a physical problem. Finding exceptions makes it easier to believe that the pain is coming from our brains and not our bodies.

If you already have some exceptions, great! If not, that's okay too. As you practice the techniques of Pain Reprocessing Therapy, you'll start discovering your own exceptions.

Building a Case

In addition to exceptions, there are other ways to get evidence that your pain isn't physically caused.

Does your pain seem to ebb and flow based on your stress level?

When your symptoms first started, did they come out of nowhere?

Has your pain persisted beyond the normal course of healing?

These signs (check out the full list in the appendix) can help you build a convincing case that your pain is neuroplastic. I encourage you to look back over your experiences to see if you can find evidence that points to neuroplastic pain.

To demonstrate the evidence-gathering process, here are the cases of two patients, Rebecca and Barry.

Rebecca

Rebecca was a college senior with a solid work ethic, a promising future, and a slightly unhealthy obsession with her dog.

A few months before graduation, Rebecca started getting pain in her wrists. It became a daily struggle, and soon she developed a conditioned response: typing. The longer she typed, the worse her pain got (not an ideal situation for a college student). She bought an ergonomic desk and keyboard, but they didn't help.

By the time she made it through finals, she was deep in the

pain-fear cycle. She spent the next couple of years terrified of typing, looking for the rare job that didn't include computer use.

When I first met with Rebecca, we started searching for evidence that her pain was neuroplastic. Unfortunately, she had no exceptions (typing *always* caused her pain), so we kept looking.

Here's what we came up with:

First, she didn't have an injury preceding the onset of pain. Her symptoms just appeared one day out of nowhere. That's very common with neuroplastic pain.

Second, the pain came on during a pretty stressful time. She was about to graduate and had no idea what she wanted to do with her life. (That is, outside of updating her dog's Instagram.)

Third, she had a history of both neck pain and knee pain. Both lasted for months. Multiple unrelated symptoms are indicative of neuroplastic pain.

Fourth, both her wrists started hurting at the same time. That's huge! Outside of an injury or disease, when two symptoms arise in mirror image of each other (both hands, both feet, etc.), that's a dead giveaway.

With these four pieces of evidence, we were able to conclude that her pain was neuroplastic.

Barry

Barry's pain started with a rather bizarre injury. He was waiting for a cab outside a bar and was randomly punched by a drunk stranger.

It cracked two of his teeth.

Even though the culprit was arrested and paid for Barry's dental bills, the damage was done. Barry developed pain in his mouth that lasted for the next six years.

Barry was determined to figure out what was causing his pain. He met with dentists, oral surgeons, and neurologists. Consequently, he was diagnosed with myofascial pain, trigeminal neuralgia, and burning mouth syndrome (yikes!).

By the time I met Barry, he'd tried every treatment imaginable, from dental splints to root canals. Understandably, it was hard for him to believe that his pain was neuroplastic—every diagnosis he'd been given and every treatment he'd received reinforced that his pain was physically caused.

So we started off by looking for evidence.

Here's what we found:

First, despite his many diagnoses, his mouth had healed. Over the years, Barry got X-rays, MRIs, and CT scans, and every image showed the same thing: there was no discernable sign of damage.

Second, his pain was a lot better in the mornings. When symptoms follow a pattern where they're better or worse depending on the time of day, that points to neuroplastic pain.

Third, there was the Tony Robbins incident.

This might be my all-time favorite piece of evidence.

A couple of years ago, Tony Robbins, the renowned motivational speaker, gave a talk at Barry's corporate retreat. The speech was so powerful, so full of hope, that Barry's pain completely disappeared! For two full weeks he was pain-free.

Though his symptoms returned, this was a huge piece of evidence. Like my Lakers game experience, the Tony Robbins incident was an exception. And it allowed us to conclude that there was nothing physically wrong with Barry's mouth.

REINFORCING THE EVIDENCE

Both Rebecca and Barry had enough evidence to determine that their pain was neuroplastic. But sometimes having conclusive evidence isn't enough.

The night of my magical Lakers experience, I remember thinking, "Now I know that my pain is neuroplastic. I'm free!" Then the following night, I went out to dinner, and as soon as I sat down, my back started hurting. It felt like my epiphany flew out the window.

No matter how much evidence we have, it can be hard to hold on to when we're in a pain state. So we don't want to just gather evidence; we want to reinforce it. Some of my patients like to make an evidence sheet—a list of all the support that shows they have neuroplastic pain. By way of example, here are the evidence sheets that Rebecca and Barry created:

REBECCA

1. Pain came out of nowhere

2. Pain came on when I was super stressed

3. Symptoms in multiple parts of my body

4. Pain started in both wrists at same time (nice try, brain!)

BARRY

1. CT scan showed that mouth is totally healed

2. Pain is better in the morning

3. No pain for two weeks after Tony Robbins talk

If you think you'd find it helpful, create your own evidence sheet. It's best to review it when you're having doubts that your pain is neuroplastic. The more you reinforce that your pain isn't dangerous, the easier it is to believe. And the more you believe, the easier it is to break out of the pain-fear cycle.

In the next chapter, I'll teach you somatic tracking, the single most powerful technique of Pain Reprocessing Therapy. It's a simple but effective skill that changes your brain's relationship with your pain.

CHAPTER 5

Somatic Tracking

The first time I watched *The Wizard of Oz*, I was captivated. The movie somehow combines tornadoes, witches, and flying monkeys. It blew my seven-year-old mind.

In the film, Dorothy and her ragtag band travel to the Emerald City, where they meet the wizard. He calls himself the Great and Powerful Oz, and he really seems great and powerful. He's a giant floating head with a booming voice, surrounded by blasts of fire. Our heroes are terrified of him, until Dorothy's adorable dog, Toto, pulls back a curtain and reveals that the wizard is just an old man using special effects to seem big and scary.

That's the plot of *The Wizard of Oz*, but it's also the plot of Pain Reprocessing Therapy. Neuroplastic pain feels great and powerful. It certainly hurts like it's great and powerful. It seems scary, like it's caused by something dangerous in your body. But it's not actually dangerous. Once we expose it as a mistake made by our brains, it loses its power. To pull the curtain back on neuroplastic pain, we need to be like Toto. We need to investigate our pain without fear. And the way we do that is called somatic tracking.

Somatic Tracking in Action

The easiest way to explain somatic tracking is with an example. So I'm going to recount a somatic tracking exercise I did with a patient named Janet. I'll take breaks along the way to describe what we did and why.

Janet had chronic back pain that had resisted all medical treatment. She'd tried physical therapy, chiropractic adjustments, and steroid injections, but nothing helped. In our first session together, I explained how the brain can misinterpret safe signals from the body as if they were dangerous ones. After reviewing the evidence, we determined that Janet had neuroplastic pain. Once Janet understood the source of her pain, she was ready for somatic tracking.

> **Me:** I know you have pain in your lower back. Does it hurt right now?
>
> **Janet:** Yes.
>
> **Me:** Okay, that's actually a good thing, because we want to explore your pain. So I'd like you to get comfortable . . . close your eyes . . . and bring your attention to your back. All we're doing is exploring the sensation of pain in your back. You don't need to get rid of the pain, you don't need to change it—you just need to observe it. How would you describe the quality of the sensation? Is it a tightness? A tingling? A warm feeling?
>
> **Janet:** It's a tight feeling . . . and it's kind of pulsing.

The first component of somatic tracking is mindfulness. Many people associate mindfulness with meditation or Eastern philosophy, but it's actually quite simple. Jon Kabat-Zinn, who helped popularize mindfulness in the West, defines it as "paying attention, on purpose, in the present moment, non-judgmentally." And that's exactly what Janet is doing here. She's paying attention to her pain, but with no agenda and no judgment.

It's not complicated, but it's very powerful. When you pay attention to your pain mindfully, you're observing it without fear. Neuroscientists have shown that mindfulness increases feelings of safety by deactivating the brain's fear circuits. This disrupts the pain-fear cycle and helps your brain interpret signals properly.

> **Me:** As you explore this tight, pulsing feeling in your back, remember that there's nothing to fear here. Neuroplastic pain is actually a safe sensation. It's just your brain overreacting to neutral, safe signals from your body.
>
> **Janet:** Okay.

Our goal is to pay attention to the pain without fear. But that can be hard when we've feared the pain for so long. The second component of somatic tracking is sending messages of safety to your brain. This technique, known as safety reappraisal, has been shown by scientists to significantly decrease fear.

Here, I'm reminding Janet that her pain is not dangerous. There's nothing to fear. It's just a misunderstanding between her brain and her body. By reinforcing that the sensation is safe, she can start to clear up the misunderstanding.

Remember the evidence you started gathering in the last

chapter? That will help you with your somatic tracking. The more evidence you collect, the more authentic and effective your messages of safety will be.

> **Me:** What do you notice happening to the sensation in your back as you focus on it? Does it intensify or subside? Does it spread out or contract? Does it move around or stay exactly the same? Does the quality of the sensation change at all?

> **Janet:** It's still pulsing, but it's spread out more. It's more diffuse now.

> **Me:** That's great. Remember, whatever happens to the sensation is okay. Because it's safe. So let it do what it's going to do. All you have to do is watch. It's like you're snorkeling or scuba diving, and you're floating there, and you see a school of beautiful fish. You're not trying to chase the fish. You're not trying to catch the fish. You're just calmly watching them. Your back is the ocean, and the sensations you're feeling are those fish. All you have to do is observe. I'm just a friendly sea turtle swimming nearby. A friendly, talking sea turtle. Okay, I may have taken this analogy too far.

This is the third component of somatic tracking. Yoni, who ran the Boulder Back Pain Study and loves fancy scientific terms, calls it "positive affect induction." I call it "making jokes." Picturing me as a talking turtle is a little silly, and that's the point. This is all about mood. We want to observe our physical sensations with lightness and curiosity.

Paying attention with lightness is an important component of somatic tracking. Scientists study positive affect by having subjects look at happy images, watch funny videos, or listen to joyful music. Experiments like this show that when people's moods are lightened, they are better at overcoming pain-related fear.

I used humor to keep Janet's mood light and relaxed, but I don't expect you to tell yourself jokes. It's not about making yourself laugh; it's about the way you look at these inner sensations. We'll talk more about cultivating this positive, curious attitude later on in the chapter.

> **Me:** You're just watching your back to see what happens. You're just an observer. These are completely safe sensations. Your brain may misinterpret them as pain sometimes, but they are safe. What do you notice happening in your back?
>
> **Janet:** It's not pulsing anymore. It's steadier. And still more spread out. It hurts less than before.
>
> **Me:** That's great, but just remember, that's not our goal. Whatever happens to the pain happens. You're just watching and feeling with lightness and curiosity. This reinforces to your brain that the sensation is safe. Now take a final few seconds to explore the sensations in your back and . . . open your eyes.

In this session, Janet was able to pay attention to her pain but through a new lens. In the past, Janet reacted to her pain with fear, which kept her stuck in the pain-fear cycle. When she did somatic tracking, Janet was able to explore her pain through a lens of safety. This is the first step in rewiring her brain to interpret the sensations from her back properly.

"Safety" is our watchword. I want you to always keep safety in mind as you do your own somatic tracking. Every component of somatic tracking is designed to reduce feelings of danger and foster a sense of safety. Mindfulness is a way to view your pain without judgment or fear. Safety reappraisal reminds your brain that these sensations aren't dangerous. And a playful mood allows you to explore the sensations in a safe, curious way.

Now It's Your Turn

Now that you've seen somatic tracking in action and you understand its components, let's give it a try. We're going to talk more about how and when to do somatic tracking later, but I'd like you to experience it firsthand. So for now, you're just going to dip your toe in to try it out.

One quick note before we get started: The goal of somatic tracking is to change your brain's relationship with your pain, so it's helpful if you experience a little pain during the exercise. (Yes, this is the one time when you actually want to have pain.) So if you have pain when you sit, do somatic tracking while sitting. If you have pain when you stand, do it standing up. If you have pain when you walk, try it while walking around.

You may find it helpful to close your eyes during somatic tracking to make it easier to focus on your inner sensations. But if you're walking around, please keep your eyes open. You can't teach your brain that it's safe if you bang your shin on the coffee table.

What I'd like you to try, for just a few moments, is to bring your attention to the sensation of pain wherever you feel it in your body.

As you explore your pain, the first thing I'd like you to do is identify the quality of the sensation. What does it feel like? Is it a tight sensation? A burning sensation? A tingling sensation? Take a few moments to check it out.

Once you've identified the quality of the sensation, explore it a little. Is it widespread, or is it localized? Does it feel the same everywhere, or is it stronger in some spots than others?

As you start to get the lay of the land, simply observe the sensation. You don't need to get rid of it, you don't need to change it—all you need to do is watch, noticing and exploring from a place of lightness and curiosity. Here's a quick dose of lightness to help you:

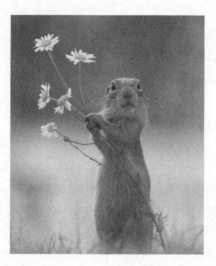

As you pay attention to the sensation in your body, what do you notice? Does it intensify? Does it subside? Does it change in quality? Does it move around? Whatever it does is okay. Remember, this is a safe sensation. It's simply your brain misinterpreting safe messages that are coming from your body. So just sit back and enjoy the show.

Take a few more seconds to explore these physical sensations with no judgment and no agenda. And . . . we're done.

Congratulations! You just did your first somatic tracking

exercise. Somewhere along the way, your brain mistakenly learned that certain sensations from your body are dangerous. Through somatic tracking, your brain will reprocess these signals and associate them with safety.

When you start doing somatic tracking on your own, having the right mindset is important. Here are two guidelines to help set you up for success: turning down the intensity and outcome independence.

TURNING DOWN THE INTENSITY

It can be challenging to track the painful sensations in your body with lightness and curiosity. Pain hurts, and chronic pain sufferers have a long and emotional relationship with their pain. This can lead to what I call "hawk mode."

When I first began leading patients in somatic tracking exercises, I noticed a common theme. While paying attention to their pain, many of them looked at it with intensity and a laser focus. They watched it like a hawk. And nothing about a hawk's burning gaze says safety.

But there's another way to pay attention. A less intense way. Like when you're enjoying a colorful sunset or lying in a field watching the clouds drift by overhead. You're still observing, but with a sense of effortlessness and curiosity. That's the kind of lightness that we want to bring to somatic tracking. I've had many patients tell me that once they paid attention to their pain with genuine curiosity, that's when somatic tracking finally clicked for them.

Remember the climactic scene from *The Wizard of Oz*: Dorothy, the Scarecrow, the Tin Man, and the Cowardly Lion are all tracking the wizard with intensity. Sometimes they're scared of him, and sometimes they're angry, but they're always intense. Meanwhile, Toto has zero intensity. He's just a curious pup, sniffing around. "Sniff, sniff, sniff. Ooh, what's that? A curtain? I love curtains! I'm gonna run in there! Hey, there's a human in here! I love humans! I'm gonna pull on this curtain and see what happens. Pulling on stuff is the best!"

Everyone else's intensity kept them stuck, feeling like they were in danger. Toto's lightness and curiosity allowed him to explore and show that the danger was an illusion, that they were actually safe. So if you find yourself tracking with intensity, try to let go of your inner hawk and tap into your inner Toto.

OUTCOME INDEPENDENCE

From 1958 to 1960, my dad was on the gymnastics team at Michigan State University. He was one of the best high-bar specialists in the country, but he had an archrival who was just as good: Abie Grossfeld.

Abie and my dad were always pushing each other to new heights. My dad would blow everyone away with a double somersault, and then Abie would come right back with an inverted giant. They were like the Bill Gates and Steve Jobs of college gymnastics.

One day at a gymnastics meet in Chicago, my dad decided to try one of the most dangerous tricks imaginable: the hop to eagle. This trick involves letting go of the bar when you're upside down and catching it a second later with a different grip.

Best-case scenario, you make history. Worst-case scenario, you *are* history.

With ten thousand fans cheering him on, my dad stepped to the mat. Halfway through his routine, he was upside down, and he went for it.

He let go of the bar.

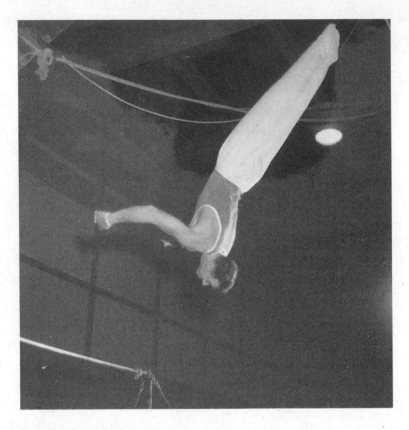

Stan Gordon, 1959

And a second later, he reached back out for it, and ... it wasn't there. My dad missed the bar completely. He went crashing to the ground as the crowd let out an audible gasp.

As my dad hobbled back to the bench, he felt a little disappointed. But there was an even stronger feeling. He felt proud. He felt bold. He may not have landed the hop to eagle, but he gave it his best shot.

That's outcome independence—when we're able to feel successful regardless of the outcome. The doing is more important than the result. And we want to approach somatic tracking the same way.

The first time I tried somatic tracking with my own pain, I was outcome independent by accident. I remember feeling a dull burning sensation in my lower back, so I just started watching it. Even though it was an unpleasant feeling, I reminded myself that it was safe and that there was nothing wrong with my body.

As I continued to observe the pain, it started to change. First it intensified, then it subsided a little, then it morphed from a burning sensation to a stabbing sensation. And then it changed again to a tingling sensation.

What was happening?

I started marveling at the power of my brain. Was I a Jedi? How was I doing this? I continued to explore. I had no desired outcome. I was just curiously watching to see what would happen next. I was actually enjoying the experience.

And then an amazing thing happened. The pain went away! I still felt a sensation in my back, but it was no longer unpleasant; it was just neutral. At long last I found a tool to get rid of my pain—or so I thought.

The next time my back hurt, I tried somatic tracking. But this time something was different. I had a clear goal: I wanted the pain to go away. I was no longer exploring the sensation with authentic curiosity. I was no longer enjoying the experience. I was frustrated and impatient and definitely not feeling like a Jedi. And the pain persisted.

In the first instance of somatic tracking, I was outcome independent. I wasn't concerned with the result, I was simply exploring with curiosity while communicating messages of safety. The second time, I was using somatic tracking as a means to an end. I wanted to get rid of the pain.

And the harder we try to get rid of our pain, the more we reinforce that it's dangerous.

Does this mean you shouldn't want your pain to go away? Of course you should! I wrote this book to help you accomplish exactly that. But there's a difference between a short-term goal and a long-term goal.

For example, when my dad missed the hop to eagle on that fateful day in Chicago, he was proud of himself just for trying. But he still wanted to win the NCAA championship down the road. Being outcome independent at smaller gymnastics meets allowed him to practice tricks without pressure and without judgment. As a result, he got better. And he ended up winning two national championships in a row. (Which he's not shy about sharing with anyone who'll listen. In fact, his personalized license plate says IINCAA. Subtle, Dad.)

The same strategy works when you practice somatic tracking. By being outcome independent, you reinforce to your brain that the pain is safe. Eventually, your brain will learn this lesson and your pain will fade. Outcome independence in the short term helps you achieve the long-term goal of eliminating your pain.

I've noticed that when my patients first start practicing somatic tracking, outcome independence can be tricky. You may struggle with it at first too. That's okay. With time and practice it gets easier.

Patient Perspective

When I first started doing somatic tracking, it was very foreign to me. It was hard because focusing on my lower back always meant immediately trying to solve the problem. I'd think, "What stretch do I need to do to undo this spasm?" Or, "Should I try the ice pack?" All my attention was oriented toward how do I undo it. So it didn't come easy to just sit there and purely observe what was going on.

One thing that helped with somatic tracking was changing the language that I used. When I thought of it as "pain," that felt like something I needed to get rid of. I started thinking of it as just "a sensation," and that helped me feel like I didn't have to fix it.

Another thing that helped was just teasing out what adjectives I would use to describe the sensation in my back. Does it feel hot or cold or spiky or pulling or poking? For whatever reason, spending time teasing out those little adjectives was helpful for me in enabling that observation process.

More and more, I was able to do somatic tracking with an inquisitive attitude. After that, the sensations became less threatening, and the pain eventually subsided.

I even started being less of a problem solver in other areas of my life. I used to focus all my energy into trying to fix every tiny issue with my relationship or my work . . . Now I'm kind of like, "You know what, let's just sit with it. It is what it is." Not having to fix everything right away is really liberating.

I've actually gotten to a place where I'm grateful that I had pain. Without it, I don't think I would have had this opportunity to take a pause and examine how I was approaching my life. But I wouldn't necessarily want to repeat it tomorrow!

–YOLANDA

You Got to Know When to Track 'Em

I'm not a big country music fan, but there's one song I've always loved: "The Gambler," most famously sung by Kenny Rogers. It tells the story of meeting a gambler "on a train bound for nowhere." In exchange for some whiskey and a cigarette (it's a country song after all), the gambler offers some advice:

> You've got to know when to hold 'em,
>
> know when to fold 'em,
>
> know when to walk away,
>
> and know when to run.
>
> You never count your money
>
> when you're sittin' at the table,
>
> there'll be time enough for countin'
>
> when the dealin's done.

The gambler was talking about poker (or more generally, life), but Kenny Rogers may as well have been singing about somatic tracking.

Somatic tracking is a powerful tool for overcoming pain. But having this tool is not enough. The key is knowing when to use somatic tracking and when to back off. In chapter 6, I'll teach you a system for practicing somatic tracking designed to maximize its effectiveness and minimize setbacks. Let's dive into "the Process."

CHAPTER 6

The Process

The Philadelphia 76ers have a rich history. Some of the greatest basketball players of all time wore the 76ers uniform: Wilt Chamberlain, Julius Erving, Charles Barkley. But lately, history is the only thing Philadelphia fans have. The 76ers haven't won an NBA championship since 1983.

A few years back, Philadelphia hired an analyst named Sam Hinkie as their new general manager. Hinkie had a controversial strategy for building a championship team. He knew that if you want to win, you need the best players. And if you want to get the best players, you need the highest picks in the annual NBA draft. So, how do you get the top draft picks?

You need to lose.

The teams with the worst records get the highest draft picks. So Sam Hinkie's bold plan was to lose. Badly. For several years in a row. Some were skeptical that Hinkie's strategy would work. One sportswriter called Hinkie "a fraud," "a dunce," and "a moron"—all in the same article! But Hinkie was undeterred. He asked 76ers fans to be patient. This was a long-term process that required trust.

So he traded away all of Philadelphia's best players. And then he traded away all of their mediocre players. And the team was bad. Very, very bad. In 2014, they broke the NBA record for consecutive losses. Then in 2015, they broke that record.

But the fans said to themselves, "Trust the process."

Time passed and Hinkie's plan started to work. Philadelphia drafted some great new players. But one of their top draft picks broke his foot and was out for a year. And then another one of their top draft picks broke *his* foot and was out for *two* years!

And the fans said, "Trust the process."

Finally, in 2017, everything started coming together. The 76ers had acquired a lot of new talent, their stars were finally healthy, and they started to win. They won five games in a row. And then ten in a row. And then fifteen!

For years, loyal Philadelphia fans had consoled themselves by wistfully murmuring, "Trust the process." But they weren't murmuring anymore. As the 76ers started winning games, their arena was filled with the deafening sound of twenty thousand fans chanting in unison, "TRUST . . . THE . . . PROCESS!"

Philadelphia ended the season with more wins than they'd had in seventeen years. But they never could have done it if they didn't have trust when things were at their worst.

Later in the chapter, I'm going to teach you a process for overcoming neuroplastic pain. It's a set of strategies that vary based on your level of pain intensity. During the Process, there will be ups and downs. Sometimes you'll feel like you're on the right track, and sometimes you may have doubts. But stay the course, like the resilient fans of the Philadelphia 76ers did. When things are at their worst, Trust the Process.

Of course, before you can Trust the Process, you need to understand why it works.

Facing Fears

As we discussed earlier, neuroplastic pain is a mistake. It's the result of your brain interpreting signals from your body as if they're dangerous. And your fear around the pain reinforces these messages of danger. So we need to address that fear.

If you want to overcome any fear, you need one thing: exposure to the thing you're afraid of. For example, if you want to overcome a fear of public speaking, you need to give speeches. If you're afraid of heights, you have to go up in tall buildings. If you're scared of conflict, come to my parents' house on Thanksgiving.

To overcome the fear of neuroplastic pain, you need exposure to the pain itself. Obviously, if you have chronic pain, you get plenty of that already, but what you need is a special kind of exposure. This is where somatic tracking comes in. By bringing your attention to the pain in a safe way, you're getting the exposure you need to overcome fear and rewire your brain.

But exposure can be a double-edged sword. When you face the thing you're scared of, it can reduce your fear, but it can also increase it. Let's start off by talking about when exposure goes well.

CORRECTIVE EXPERIENCES

A few years ago, my friend Phil adopted a dog named Rocky from a shelter. Rocky was very sweet, but he'd been treated poorly for the first few years of his life, so he was a bundle of nerves. Whenever there was a knock at the door, Rocky would run and cower behind the couch. Because he'd been mistreated, he had learned that people = danger. Poor pup.

All Phil's friends knew about Rocky's fear. So every time we came over, we'd make a special effort to treat Rocky nicely. We'd use gentle voices and avoid sudden movements, and once Rocky was ready, we'd give him lots of ear scratches and belly rubs.

Each time Rocky interacted with a stranger in a way that made him feel safe, it helped reduce his fear. This is called a "corrective experience." After many corrective experiences, Rocky was able to unlearn his fear and replace it with a new association: people = safe. Eventually, instead of hiding behind the couch when he heard a knock, Rocky would rush to the door, eager to greet visitors.

If you feel safe during exposure to the source of your fear, it's a corrective experience. And this is the path to overcoming neuroplastic pain. With enough corrective experiences, your brain will learn that the signals coming from your body are, in fact, safe.

But if you confront the thing you're afraid of in a way that makes you feel danger, it can reinforce your fear.

SETBACKS

When we got the opportunity to do the Boulder Back Pain Study, I knew that I couldn't treat all the patients by myself. I needed help, and Christie was the perfect choice. We've worked together for years, she's an expert in Pain Reprocessing Therapy, and her patients love her. There was just one problem: Christie is scared of flying.

Christie bravely agreed to face her fear, and I gave her some encouragement:

> **Me:** Flying back and forth between L.A. and Colorado will actually be a good thing. You'll have so many opportunities for corrective experiences!
>
> **Christie:** Great . . .

And for the first few trips, I was right. Until one fateful flight back to L.A.

Christie boarded with a sense of optimism. The flights had all gone smoothly so far. As she sat in the middle seat, Christie said hello to the woman sitting next to her. They never exchanged names, so I'll just call her Doomsday Donna, for reasons that will become clear.

> **Doomsday Donna:** You know, they just retired this type of airplane. This is probably the last flight for this plane. I hope we make it back to L.A.
>
> **Christie:** What?!

It turns out that Doomsday Donna was even more scared of flying than Christie was. And Doomsday Donna wasn't shy about sharing her fears with anyone who would listen. Was the plane really about to be retired? Who knows? Christie had no time for fact-checking. The plane was taking off, and so was Christie's anxiety.

Christie spent the rest of the flight attempting relaxation exercises, giving herself messages of safety, and avoiding eye contact with Doomsday Donna. But as they made their final approach into LAX, they heard an unusual grinding sound coming from the bottom of the plane.

Doomsday Donna: I think there's a problem with the landing gear.

Christie: No, I'm sure it's fi–

Doomsday Donna: I think the wheels are stuck inside the plane. We're going to land without landing gear!

Christie: *Whimper.*

In retrospect, it's obvious that Doomsday Donna didn't know what she was talking about. But by this point, Christie was in a full-blown panic, so she wasn't exactly thinking logically. She was too busy imagining an emergency water landing and cursing herself for not having studied the safety card in her seatback pocket.

As the plane hurtled toward the earth, Christie's fingernails sank deeper and deeper into her armrests. Just when Christie (and the armrests) couldn't take it anymore, the plane touched down. On land. On its fully functioning wheels. The flight was over, but the damage was done. Christie was a mess. She couldn't speak a single word for forty-five minutes.

Needless to say, this was not a corrective experience. Christie definitely exposed herself to her fear, but unfortunately in a way that made her feel less safe. Exposure with a sense of safety leads to a corrective experience. But when exposure triggers feelings of danger, the fear gets stronger. Since that's the opposite of what we want to happen, we call it a setback. That's okay. Setbacks will happen. They are temporary. After her setback, Christie continued working on her fear of flying. She was patient, collected more corrective experiences, and stopped talking to the people sitting next to her.

As you work your way through the Process, you will experience setbacks sometimes. All pain sufferers do.

One of my patients had a setback when he went out for burgers with some friends. He was a little worried about his pain beforehand, but he really wanted to hang out with his buddies. Unfortunately, his pain was a steady throb all through lunch, and he had a terrible time. Frustrated, he thought, "I can't even do things I enjoy without my pain ruining it!"

Another patient had been feeling pretty good for a few days in a row, until she had a stressful conversation with her son. Her pain spiked and stayed high for the next two days. She was despondent. She thought, "If even the littlest bit of stress can trigger this much pain, how am I ever going to get better?"

A third patient had a pain flare-up that seemingly came out of nowhere. It felt totally random. It really scared her because she thought that if she couldn't identify why her pain came on, then she'd never be able to stop it.

Their circumstances were all different, but in each case, the patient's fear around their pain increased. That's a setback. However, I'm happy to report that all these setbacks were temporary. All three patients trusted the Process and continued working toward recovery.

Setbacks are like speed bumps on the road to a pain-free life. They may slow you down, but as long as you stay the course, they can't stop you.

AN EXCELLENT EXPOSURE

No matter how strong a fear is, with enough corrective experiences, our brains can develop a new understanding. The way to break out of the pain-fear cycle is simply to experience your pain in a safe way. Somatic tracking is that way.

As I mentioned earlier, somatic tracking is a way of getting exposure to your pain through a lens of safety. In other words, somatic tracking is a form of exposure that's been carefully designed to create corrective experiences.

Somatic tracking is the cornerstone of Pain Reprocessing Therapy. But there's one more tool you need to navigate the Process: avoidance behaviors.

THE OPPOSITE OF EXPOSURE

When you face the source of your fear, that's exposure. When you try to escape your fear, that's avoidance behavior. When Rocky the rescue dog hid behind the couch, he was engaging in an avoidance behavior. If Christie refused to fly back to Colorado and instead took a twenty-two-hour bus ride (like she threatened to), that would be an avoidance behavior. And a totally reasonable one.

Sometimes people feel guilty for using avoidance behaviors. "Avoidance" makes it sound like you're running away from your problems. But when used strategically, avoidance behaviors are an effective tool for overcoming fear.

Avoidance behaviors are really common with chronic pain patients. Anything you do to reduce your pain (or to keep from triggering it in the first place) is an avoidance behavior. But they often vary from person to person. To give you examples of common avoidance behaviors, let's look back at some of the patients I presented in chapters 3 and 4.

- Melanie was the patient who developed chronic headaches after a lifetime of worrying. She had several avoidance behaviors that helped reduce her pain. For temporary relief, Melanie would massage her temples. But for a really bad headache, she would either lie down in the dark or take a hot bath.

- James was the patient who injured his back playing basketball (and was always behind on his emails). James's back pain was triggered by sitting, so his go-to avoidance behavior was standing up. If he had to sit for long stretches, he'd use back pillows and heating pads to reduce the pain.

- Rebecca was the college student who had hand and wrist pain when she typed. Her main avoidance behavior was taking breaks from typing. Also, she found that both stretching and cracking her wrists brought her a little relief.

- Barry was the patient who developed chronic mouth pain. He had one effective avoidance behavior: chewing mints—and the stronger the mint, the better. When he was focused on the flavor of the mint, he found that he was less aware of the pain.

When you suffer from chronic pain, avoidance behaviors become a way of life. Through trial and error, we learn how to prevent and manage our pain as much as possible. I'd like you to think about your own avoidance behaviors. What are the things that bring you relief when your pain is bad? In the next few sections, I'll teach you how to use your avoidance behaviors as part of the Process.

Putting the Pieces Together

Sometimes I play board games with my nieces. Their favorite is Chutes and Ladders. You probably played it as a kid too. It's a very simple game. You move along the board and try to reach the finish line. If you land on a space with a ladder, you get to jump ahead a few squares and you're closer to winning. When my nieces hit a ladder, they act like they just won the lottery. It's adorable. If you end up on a square with a chute, you slide backward and lose some spaces. This is less adorable, since it sometimes leads to tears and the board getting flipped over.

Pain Reprocessing Therapy works exactly the same way. Our finish line is living a pain-free life. A corrective experience is like a ladder: your brain learns that your pain is actually safe, and you move closer to the finish line. A setback is like a chute. The association between pain and danger is reinforced, and you slide a little further from the goal.

To "win" at Pain Reprocessing Therapy, we want to maximize the number of corrective experiences and minimize setbacks. To help us do that, we have two powerful tools: somatic tracking and avoidance behaviors. The Process outlines exactly how to use each tool to reach the finish line. But before I get into the nuts and bolts of the Process, here are two pieces of general advice:

First, the Process will tell you what to do and when to do it. But I don't want it to become a job or an obsession for you. Please don't approach these guidelines with a sense of pressure or urgency. Remember, pressure puts your brain on high alert. We want to practice the Process with a sense of patience and safety. I want you to enjoy your life as much as possible, knowing that if you follow the steps, your pain will eventually fade. Trust the Process!

Second, setbacks are normal. They are not a big deal, and I don't want you to be scared of them. Notice that I said our goal is to "minimize setbacks." I didn't say "eliminate setbacks," because that's impossible. Please don't worry or beat yourself up when you have a setback. Those things just make you feel bad and put your brain on high alert. I'll give you the same advice I give my nieces: "It's natural to feel disappointed when you land on a chute. I get it. I don't like chutes either. But they are part of the game, and they shouldn't keep us from having fun. There are still a ton of ladders waiting for you! And please stop hitting your sister."

Without further ado, let's dive in. The Process is based on your pain intensity. Depending on your level of pain, different strategies will help you collect corrective experiences while avoiding setbacks as much as possible.

WHEN YOUR PAIN IS HIGH

When you have high levels of pain, your brain is feeling a lot of danger. That means it's pretty much impossible to have a corrective experience. So we're not even going to attempt somatic tracking. That's okay—we'll have opportunities for corrective experiences later. In the meantime, we want to minimize setbacks as much as possible. So, when your pain is high, you want to engage in avoidance behaviors.

If you have to stand up every ten minutes or sit down every ten minutes, do it! If you have to use a pillow or a hot-water bottle or massage the body part that hurts, do it! When your pain is high, do whatever you need to do to feel more comfortable. The one thing you don't want to do is push through the pain. I learned this lesson the hard way.

One day, long before I developed the Process, my back was in a lot of pain. I was incredibly frustrated. I had collected enough evidence to know that my pain was neuroplastic, but I hadn't figured out how to get rid of it yet. I thought, "I'm going to stand up to my pain. I'm going to prove to my brain that I can sit for as long as I want!" So I got in my car, filled up the tank, stocked up on important supplies like Cool Ranch Doritos, and drove to San Francisco without stopping.

Los Angeles to San Francisco is a five-hour drive. After three hours, my back pain was a 9 out of 10. But I pushed through the pain.

After four hours, I had 10-out-of-10 pain. But I pushed through.

After five hours, I realized, "Oh, that wasn't 10-out-of-10 pain after all. *This* is 10-out-of-10 pain!"

I finally got to San Francisco. I was delirious from pain. I had no idea where I was. I have vague memories of a wharf. I parked, opened the car door, and fell on the ground. And I just lay there, filled with pain. And regret. And Doritos.

I wanted to teach my brain a lesson, and I did. Unfortunately, I taught my brain that my pain was even more dangerous than I'd thought before. It was a setback of epic proportions.

Sometimes we think it's empowering to push through when our pain is high, but it's the opposite. Pushing through will lead to a setback. When you fight against your pain, you are just putting your brain on high alert and reinforcing that the pain is dangerous.

When your pain is high, you may already be engaging in as

many avoidance behaviors as possible. If so, that's great. If not, now is the time to start. Either way, there's another component to this part of the Process.

When your pain is high, your brain is flooded with danger. Because of this, it's common to have thoughts of fear and hopelessness:

"I'm never going to get out of pain."

"This process isn't going to work for me."

"I'm doomed."

I could fill a whole journal with the terrifying and hopeless thoughts I had when my pain was at its worst. It's hard not to have these types of thoughts when we're in a high state of suffering. But the truth is that these types of thoughts send us even deeper into a state of fear.

Imagine a child during his first thunderstorm. The flashes of lightning and loud crashes are already scaring him. Now imagine telling that child, "Uh-oh, this is probably the apocalypse!"

That kid goes from feeling scared to feeling terrified. What he really needs more than anything is soothing. A calm, strong voice telling him that he's safe, that the storm will pass, and that he's going to be okay.

And that is exactly what you need when your pain is high. So, in addition to engaging in avoidance behaviors, you want to send yourself messages of safety. These messages can be anything that makes you feel safe. The goal is to help calm your high-alert state. Here are some examples that have worked for my patients:

- "This is temporary. I'm going to be okay."
- "I'm safe, and my body is fine."

- "My brain thinks I'm in danger, but it's just a false alarm."
- And of course: "Trust the Process."

The words themselves don't matter as much as the spirit behind the words does. Your brain is feeling danger, and you're calming it with messages of safety. This is a big part of breaking the pain-fear cycle.

You may not be able to practice avoidance behaviors all the time. And you may not be able to give yourself messages of safety all the time. But use them as much as possible to make this difficult period more tolerable and minimize setbacks.

WHEN YOUR PAIN IS LOW OR MODERATE

When you have low or medium levels of pain, you can still engage in avoidance behaviors; it's always okay to feel more comfortable if you can. But now that your pain is more tolerable, you have the opportunity to get some corrective experiences with somatic tracking. Remember, we don't want to be obsessive about it. This shouldn't be intense or urgent. You want it to be easy and effortless. You might think, "Oh cool, my pain is only like a 2 out of 10. This is a good chance to try somatic tracking."

If your pain changes or moves or decreases while you're tracking it, that's fine. But a successful corrective experience doesn't mean the pain goes away. That's our long-term goal, but right now, we're just reinforcing that the pain isn't dangerous. And we do that by tracking without trying to change anything, and without intensity. The goal is to feel good. "Hey, I just got a little exposure and I feel okay!"

My patients always have the same two questions about this part of the Process:

1. How long should each somatic tracking session be?

Think about the first time you rode a bike. It's a new activity, and it takes some getting used to. At first, you're able to stay upright for only a few seconds before hopping off. But with practice, you're able to ride around for longer and longer.

I recommend the same approach with somatic tracking. Start small. Gradually make your sessions longer. If you find yourself straining or it gets too painful, then stop.

I had a patient who could do somatic tracking for only one second at first! We tried two seconds, and it became difficult for her to tolerate. That's okay. She did it for one second at a time until she felt comfortable going for longer.

Listen to your body. If you're exploring your pain with curiosity and lightness, feel free to keep going. If it feels like a chore or is becoming intense, it's time to stop. You know you're doing somatic tracking right when it feels relaxing and safe and good.

Once you get a little experience with somatic tracking, you can determine what works best for you. Of course, you don't have to do it for longer just because you can. Some of my patients like practicing for five minutes; others like doing five-second check-ins and getting back to their day.

2. How often should I do somatic tracking?

There is no one-size-fits-all answer for this. Some of my patients want me to give them rigid rules and specific schedules. I tell them that quality is more important than quantity. The goal is to enjoy your life as much as possible while snatching a corrective experience here and there.

When I first started practicing somatic tracking, it was very regimented—several times a day for five minutes per session. This approach didn't work for me. It felt like a job, something I *had* to do and something I felt guilty about if I didn't do it enough.

So I changed it up. I began practicing somatic tracking when I was out in the world just living my life. Maybe I'd be driving to the grocery store, enjoying the day. If the pain wasn't too bad, I'd check in with it for a bit, and then I'd get back to what I was doing. Some days I'd do it half a dozen times, while some days I wouldn't do it at all.

Once I took the pressure off, somatic tracking became kind of fun. I did it when I wanted to and for as long as I felt like it.

How often you do somatic tracking is less important than the mindset and spirit with which you do it. You know yourself best. If you're the kind of person who tends to go overboard, if you are starting to obsess about doing somatic tracking, then dial it back. If you are truly enjoying somatic tracking, then go ahead and do it as much as you want.

WHEN YOU HAVE NO PAIN

When you don't have any symptoms, you're not getting any exposure to the pain. So you can't get any corrective experiences, and you're not susceptible to setbacks. But is there something you can do during these times to help overcome your symptoms? Of course there is. There are still things you can do to reduce your overall level of fear. But we'll get to those in chapters 7 and 8.

Patient Perspective

Forever is the scariest thing. That's what I was most afraid of. The thought of living in pain for the rest of my life was unbearable. And that definitely impacted my recovery.

When I first started the treatment, I saw results pretty quickly. The pain was lower, and I was able to do more and more. But after a little bit, the pain came back, and it terrified me. I'd been doing so well—why was I going backward?!

I felt very out of control. I thought if I worked harder and did more somatic tracking, it could help. I started doing somatic tracking morning, afternoon, and night.

I'm the type of person that if you give me a method, I'm going to keep at it until it works. That's what I was trying to do. But it was too much. I overdid it. Without even realizing it, I was obsessing.

Then I realized that I was trying too hard to get rid of the pain, and it was just generating more stress. I needed to change my approach.

I started doing somatic tracking less often. But more important, I started doing it differently. Instead of looking at it as a chore, I saw it as a way to take care of myself. A way to make myself feel safe.

As I became less afraid of the pain, it started decreasing. I had hope again. I knew there would be ups and downs, good days and bad days, but I had learned how to handle them.

Nowadays I still get a little pain occasionally, but it doesn't scare me anymore. Sometimes after a stressful day at work, I'll feel tightness in my neck and shoulders, but I know not to panic. I know how to deal with it now. And I know it's not forever.

—GRACE

As You Go Through the Process

Now you have a set of strategies to navigate your symptoms based on your level of pain intensity. However, the Process isn't linear. You may have a lot of pain in the morning, no pain in the afternoon, and more again at night. That's okay. The pattern of the pain is less important than the way you respond.

Whether your pain is high, medium, or low, you have a set of guidelines to help you through it. And you're teaching your brain to feel safe in the best way you can in any given moment.

OPPORTUNITY KNOCKS

We have a tendency to get excited when the pain is gone and disappointed when it returns. This makes all the sense in the world. Pain feels terrible, so of course we're going to be upset when it intensifies. But as natural as this reaction is, it brings us right back into the pain-fear cycle.

It can be helpful to change our perspective about the onset of pain. To actually look at it as an opportunity. As you know, the only way to get corrective experiences is through exposure. Each corrective experience teaches your brain that these sensations are actually safe. So one way of looking at it is that every time you have pain, it's an opportunity to rewire your brain.

Some of my patients get so good at corrective experiences that they actually start to look forward to having pain. They develop an empowered attitude of "Bring it on!" I know, I know. It sounds crazy. When you have chronic pain, so much of your life is devoted to trying to escape the pain that it's hard to imagine someone welcoming it. But it's true.

One of my favorite empowerment stories involves a patient

named Daisy. She had struggled with low back pain for six years when she started treatment. One of her most consistent pain triggers was bending over. This was particularly disastrous because Daisy is a yoga instructor!

Daisy really embraced somatic tracking and the Process. As the weeks went by, she had more and more corrective experiences. Her pain was getting lower, and her confidence was high. Her fear was definitely on the way out. But because her pain had diminished, she didn't have many opportunities to do somatic tracking. So she would actually get excited when she would feel something in her back and have a chance to go for a corrective experience.

One day, Daisy texted me: "I was gardening for 3 hours today and I only got 2 chances to do somatic tracking." She was disappointed that in a full afternoon of bending over in her yard, she'd only had two twinges of pain. That's empowerment!

The empowered approach isn't for everyone. There's no need to force it if it isn't your style. It needs to be authentic. Many of my patients have gotten out of pain without taking a "bring it on" approach.

But if taking an empowered stance does resonate with you, you may even want to seek out opportunities for somatic tracking. For example, if walking is a trigger for your pain, you could take a stroll around your neighborhood. And though I love an empowered approach, you should still take it slow. Don't sign up for a marathon just yet.

EXTINCTION BURSTS

For many pain patients, just as their fear decreases, just as their symptoms start abating, just as they begin making some real progress—*pow!* They get blindsided by intense pain. This, of course, terrifies them, and they get sucked right back into the pain-fear cycle.

To understand this phenomenon, we need to go back about eighty years to a Harvard psychologist named B. F. Skinner. Skinner studied how behaviors are learned. He did all kinds of fascinating experiments, once even teaching a couple of pigeons to play Ping-Pong.

His most notable experiment involved placing a rat inside an enclosed chamber. When the rat pressed a lever, a food pellet was released. Naturally, the rat learned to press the lever whenever it was hungry. But then one day, there was an unexpected twist—the contraption broke. A rat pressed the lever, and the pellet dispenser jammed. Instead of a snack, the rat got nothing. Eventually, the rat stopped pressing the lever. No behavior continues if it's not getting reinforced. This is called extinction. Just like the dinosaurs, the behavior died out.

But before the rat gave up, an interesting thing happened: it pressed the lever like crazy. Over and over and over it pressed, hoping that if it were persistent enough, it would get a delicious rat pellet.

This is called an extinction burst. Behaviors don't give up without a fight.

By authentically changing your relationship with fear, you can start breaking out of the pain-fear cycle, and your symptoms will begin to fade. But if fear has been part of your life for a long time, your brain has become accustomed to it, and it may not go quietly.

Many of my patients experience an extinction burst as a flare-up of their original pain. A smaller number experience it as a new type of pain. In the Boulder Back Pain Study, a few people had extinction bursts in which the pain moved to their foot or knee or hips.

Whether it's the old pain trying to make a comeback or brand-new pain, the solution is the same: stay the course. Don't fall back into the fear trap—just keep doing what you're doing. Keep applying the techniques of the Process and teaching your brain that it's safe. The burst will pass.

An extinction burst can be scary if you're not ready for it, but when you understand it, you know that it's nothing to fear. In fact, it can even be a positive sign. After all, extinction bursts only happen during extinction. So if you experience one, just tell yourself, "I'm on the right track. This is a sign that my pain is on its way out!"

The Process in Action

In the last two chapters, I've covered somatic tracking, the Process, exposure, corrective experiences, setbacks, avoidance behaviors, and extinction bursts. I know it's a lot. I think it's helpful to see how all these pieces fit together. So here's the case study of a patient named Hannah and her full experience with Pain Reprocessing Therapy.

Hannah was one of my patients in the Boulder Back Pain Study. She'd had pain in her sacrum area (where the back meets the pelvis) for more than a decade. Her pain would range from a 2 out of 10 all the way up to a 9 out of 10. Over the years, she saw various medical professionals and received various diagnoses. Hannah was told that she had ligament laxity (loose ligaments), that her hips were rotating too much, that one leg was shorter than the other, and that she had scoliosis. Sheesh! Hannah is a healthy, active woman, but all these diagnoses made her feel like a broken-down pile of floppy ligaments and twisted bones.

One of Hannah's main pain triggers was walking. Based on all her diagnoses, she constructed a scenario of what she imagined was happening in her body: "When I walk, I rotate my hips too much, and my sacrum slips out of place and gets jammed." No wonder walking caused her so much pain. Imagining that her bones were moving and jamming filled her with a huge amount of fear.

Hannah had two other pain triggers in addition to walking. One, sitting in chairs where the seat was lower than her knees (like the driver's seat of her car) consistently caused her pain. In fact, she called herself "Pillow Girl" because she was always dragging around pillows to sit on. And two, standing aggravated her back. This was pretty inconvenient, because Hannah is a teacher who stands at the front of a class for hours a day.

Hannah had a lot of frustration around her pain, which is totally reasonable. Sometimes she was angry at the pain. Sometimes she was even angry at the furniture. (She once told me, "There's a chair in my house that's too low for me to sit in. I'm very mad about that chair.") But mostly, Hannah was angry at herself. Hannah blamed herself for her pain. She confessed to me, "It's been ten years. I should have figured this out by now." In addition to her fear, Hannah clearly put a lot of pressure on herself, which contributed to her high-alert state.

In our first session, I explained how neuroplastic pain works and how the pain-fear cycle keeps us trapped. Hannah had believed her pain was caused by structural problems for a long time, but she agreed to keep an open mind.

I taught Hannah how to do somatic tracking. I explained the rules of the Process to her. I told her that when her pain was high, she should engage in as many avoidance behaviors as possible. She should minimize her walking, sit on a tall chair or stool when she was teaching, and use as many pillows as her heart desired. But when her pain was lower, I encouraged her to use somatic tracking to get some corrective experiences.

The next time she came in for a session, she was in pain and even more frustrated than before. "Alan, I'm not doing somatic tracking right!" (I told you she was hard on herself.) So we talked about what she'd been doing, and it was clear that she'd been tracking with intensity. She was extremely frustrated, and that made it difficult to track with lightness and curiosity. She told me that she felt like she was "doing battle with the pain." Hannah was trying to use somatic tracking as a weapon instead of as a tool. She wasn't just watching the pain like a hawk; she wanted to rip it to shreds like a hawk. By fighting against the pain, she was accidentally reinforcing that it was dangerous.

Hannah needed a fresh start. We decided to leave the office and go outside. It was a beautiful Colorado day. We walked around the parking lot and enjoyed the sun on our faces. She did a quick somatic tracking exercise and was finally able to let go of her intensity. At least temporarily, she wasn't doing battle with the pain. That allowed her to do somatic tracking in an effortless way. She told me, "For the first time, I was noticing instead of fixing."

Following this success, I encouraged her to keep trying to do somatic tracking with her newfound lightness. Before, she had been trying to do somatic tracking for five minutes at a time. Now she dialed it way back to five seconds at a time. Sometimes she had corrective experiences. Sometimes she didn't. But with practice, she got better. Her somatic tracking sessions became less intense. Then they started to get longer. Her brain started developing a new, safer understanding of the sensations from her body. Her pain was lower than it had been in ten years.

And then came the hike.

Toward the end of the study, Hannah, feeling confident, went on a long hike (8.4 miles, to be exact). By the time she got home, her back was screaming in 9-out-of-10 pain. It was a terrible extinction burst.

Hannah was devastated. She was frustrated with me and with the treatment. She said that she "was ready to throw the whole damn thing out." When the pain came back, everything came back with it: her fear, her intensity, and the pressure she put on herself. She felt as if she had failed.

After a few hours, Hannah decided she wasn't ready to give up. She made a conscious choice to Trust the Process. She told herself, "This is temporary. I know that I'm safe." Two days later, her back was just like it had been before the extinction burst.

Hannah continued using the Process and getting corrective experiences when she could. She also focused on just living her life. Eventually, her pain disappeared completely. She still has the same car with the same driver's seat, but now she sits in it without a pillow and doesn't have any pain. She's not mad at that low chair in her house anymore, because she can sit in it with no problem. She walks and hikes for long distances and her back is fine.

Six months after the study finished, this is what Hannah had to say about her experience:

> *This treatment was life transforming for me. During the study, Alan once asked me, "Are you willing to embrace the notion that you could be a pain-free person?" And I said no! It was outside what I could imagine. I'd been in pain for so long, I couldn't even picture that.*
>
> *Now I feel like I've transformed from an old identity into a new one. I had to disidentify from the pain. And all the fear and shame that came with it. Once I stopped trying so hard to rid myself of the pain, it freed me up to enjoy my life.*

Now It's Your Turn

I'm thrilled to tell you that you are ready to start treating your own pain. You learned about pain and fear and the amazing power of your brain. You tried out somatic tracking, and you're ready to start using it while following the rules of the Process.

Like Hannah, you may have good times and hard times. Some of these techniques are intuitive. Others take more practice. I've said it before and I'll say it again: Trust the Process. But also trust yourself. No one knows you like you. I've tried to explain not just the techniques of Pain Reprocessing Therapy but also the meaning behind them. Since you understand the goals, you can forge your own path. If something is making you feel calm and safe, by all means keep doing it. If something is causing fear or pain, take a break. This isn't about following the rules to the letter or pressuring yourself to be perfect. This is about gradually and gently teaching your brain a new path.

I hope this doesn't sound like a goodbye speech, because I still have more to share with you. So far, we've been focused on using safety to target your pain directly. But pain doesn't arise in a vacuum. In the next chapter, I'll show you how to increase your overall sense of safety to improve your pain and your life.

CHAPTER 7

Breaking the High-Alert Habit

Rachel rushed into my office like a whirlwind. "I'm so sorry I'm late!" she exclaimed as she flopped into a chair. Rachel, a high-powered executive, had been struggling with headaches for years. She'd been a patient for only a few weeks, but this was already her standard entrance. We chatted for a little bit, and she told me about the symptoms she'd had in the past week.

> **Me:** Last time, we talked about the importance of fear. I told you how it puts your brain on high alert, which can lead to pain.
>
> **Rachel:** Yeah, I've been thinking about that, but I don't really think I have fear.
>
> **Me:** Well, let me ask you this: How did you feel when you were driving here today?
>
> **Rachel:** Umm, I was rushing because I didn't want to be late. I promised myself I would be on time this week, but I got an

important email right before I was leaving, and I had to respond right away.

Me: I understand. And how many times have you checked your email today?

Rachel: Well, I had to put out a bunch of fires . . . Maybe fifty times?

Me: Gotcha. Last question: As you were driving here today and you were rushing because you were running late, did you check your email in the car?

Rachel: Well . . . yeah, but only at red lights, so it wasn't dangerous or anything!

Me: So just to sum up: So far today you've been putting out fires and rushing to not be late. It's not even noon yet, and you've checked your email more than fifty times, including in the car on the way here. And you don't think your brain is on high alert?

Rachel: That's not high alert. That's just . . . normal.

The truth is, we were both right. Rachel's lifestyle was absolutely putting her brain on high alert. And for many of us, living in a constant state of high alert has become the new normal. In a recent study, 35 percent of people worldwide said they had stress "during a lot of the day." It's a global issue, but the United States is particularly good at it. In that same survey, a whopping 55 percent of Americans said they had a lot of stress. We had the fourth-highest score out of 143 countries. Why are we so stressed-out?

Zebra 2.0

In chapter 3, we met two zebras: Nervous Nick, who is always afraid, and Fearless Frank, who never is. But the truth is that all zebras (and humans) are capable of both extremes. We've evolved the capacity to be fearful in certain situations while being calm in others. To illustrate, let's look at a third zebra, Normal Neil.

When Normal Neil spots a lion, he's instantly on high alert. His brain triggers the release of stress hormones like adrenaline and cortisol that make his heart pump fast, send extra blood to his muscles, and give him a boost of energy. This is known as the fight-or-flight response. Neil's not much of a fighter, so he'll choose flight every time, and with the help of these hormones, he takes off like greased lightning.

The fight-or-flight response helps Neil outrun lions, but he's not on high alert all the time. Most of the time, Neil is a low-alert kind of guy who enjoys chilling with his buddies, grazing, and soaking up the African sun. Except for the occasional run-for-your-life situation, Neil's existence on the savanna is mostly calm.

But what if we gave Normal Neil some upgrades?

First, let's give Neil a TV. Now he can watch the Zebra News Network. ZNN has twenty-four-hour coverage of zebra-related news from all over the world, but it's mostly about lions. Neil watches stories about recent lion attacks, future lion attacks, and a terrifying segment called "Are Lions Getting Faster?" Even though there are no actual lions nearby, Neil is now on high alert.

Next, let's give Neil a cell phone. The African plains are quite large, so Neil uses Instagram to keep up with his 'bras who are far away. But for some reason, his zebra friends always seem like they're doing better than Neil is. Their stripes are perfectly groomed, their mates are good-looking, and the grass they're eating literally looks greener than Neil's grass. With each notification ping, Neil gets a little jolt of hormones, keeping him on high alert.

Finally, let's give Neil a job to pay for his cable and cell phone bill. Unfortunately, there are no jobs locally, so he has to commute forty-five minutes to Antelope Springs. Within a few hours of arriving, his phone's ringing off the hook, his calendar's overflowing with meetings, and the spreadsheet he's working on keeps crashing his computer. It's his first day and Neil already needs a vacation.

With just a few simple tweaks, we've turned an easygoing zebra into a panicky, insecure, overworked bundle of stress.

Lower Your Alert to Lower Your Pain

Don't get me wrong, I love the modern world. It's given us medical breakthroughs, international travel, and seventy-two different flavors of Oreos. But it's also given us a level of stimulation that's unheard of in the animal kingdom.

We're wired to seek out things that stimulate us. In the wild, these things are rare and important for survival, like nutritious food and attractive mates. In our current world, they are definitely not rare. We're constantly bombarded with emails, texts, calls, meetings, articles, ads, videos, etc. And they are definitely not important for our survival.

Because our brains are designed for that old world, it's easy to get overstimulated. And much like Rachel, whom we met at the beginning of this chapter, many of us engage in behaviors that put our brains on high alert without even realizing it.

As I explained in chapter 3, whether you call it fear or stress or overstimulation, when your brain is on high alert, it's more sensitive to pain. This might sound like bad news, since we live in a world that seems determined to keep us on high alert, but it's actually good news. Because once you recognize how you're unintentionally putting your brain on high alert, you can change it. By making simple adjustments to some of your daily behaviors, you can keep your brain in a calmer state and reduce your pain.

Less pain is always a good thing, but it will also help you with the Process. When your pain is lower, it reduces the likelihood of setbacks and makes it easier to get corrective experiences.

But just like everything else in this book, the goal is not perfection. You don't have to throw your smartphone out the window. You don't have to quit your job. You don't have to meditate on a mountaintop. All you have to do is recognize behaviors that are needlessly putting your brain on high alert and do them less. That's it! Over time, cutting back on those behaviors will calm your brain and lower your pain. But pressure and perfectionism have the opposite effect. So please be patient with yourself. It takes time to change old habits.

THE SLOT MACHINE IN YOUR POCKET

I went to elementary school with a guy named Brett. Nice guy. Good at dodgeball. I haven't talked to Brett in thirty years. And yet I know what Brett had for brunch yesterday. How do I know that? Well, Brett took a picture of his brunch, wrote "yummy nom nom" on it, and posted it to social media. Hundreds of miles away, my phone dinged to let me know that one of my friends had a new post. I clicked on it, and now I know. It was French toast. (For the record, it did look yummy nom nom.)

I know about Brett's French toast because I clicked on that notification. But why I clicked on that notification is a whole other question. And the answer has to do with rats and slot machines.

In chapter 6, I told you about B. F. Skinner and his rat experiments. Every time a rat pressed a lever, it got a food pellet. Since rats love food pellets, the behavior was reinforced and became a habit. This type of reinforcement is called "continuous," because every lever press releases a pellet. Continuous reinforcement forms pretty strong habits. But then Skinner discovered a way to make even stronger habits: intermittent reinforcement. With this type of reinforcement, sometimes when the rat pressed the lever, it got a tasty snack, but sometimes it got nothing. Intermittent reinforcement creates habits that are very difficult to break.

Skinner basically built a rat slot machine. The rats were like desperate gamblers in Las Vegas who just kept pulling that lever hoping that this time they would hit the jackpot (except without the cigarette smoke and watered-down drinks). When the rats or gamblers "win," their neurons release a chemical called dopamine, which is part of the brain's reward system. Dopamine gets triggered by things like eating food and having sex and basically makes us want to keep doing those things. In other words, dopamine creates habits. It can also create addictions—cocaine works by boosting dopamine in the brain.

Dopamine keeps gamblers gambling, but that's not the only thing going on in their brains. Gamblers also have elevated levels of one of the stress hormones we talked about earlier—cortisol. Which makes sense, because gambling is stressful! Winning is exciting, but losing is painful, and either way you're on high alert. FYI, if you have chronic pain, professional gambler is a terrible career choice.

The problem is that cell phones also make our brains release dopamine and cortisol. In a way, they're just like gambling. Every time you hear a notification ding or feel a buzz in your pocket, it's like rolling the dice. Will it be a nice text from a friend? Or an annoying work email? Did a possible soul mate swipe right on you in a dating app? Or is your alma mater hitting you up for a donation?

Scientists have found that your cortisol levels go up whenever you hear your phone or even think you hear it. (Eighty-nine percent of people in one study had experienced "phantom vibrations,"—they thought their phone was vibrating when it really wasn't. That has "high alert" written all over it.) When my phone dinged to let me know about Brett's brunch, my brain experienced a powerful cocktail of dopamine and cortisol. It gave me a jolt of high alert. And all I got out of it was a photo of some French toast that I didn't even get to nom nom. Was it worth it?

The dopamine keeps us coming back to our phones, and the cortisol keeps us on high alert. One survey in the U.K. found that the average person checks their smartphone 221 times per day. That's a lot of high alert.

This doesn't apply just to phones. If you're checking your email obsessively, watching the news all day, or getting into internet arguments repeatedly, you are putting your brain on high alert, and your pain will reflect that.

I'm not asking you to give up all modern technology. I'm simply suggesting that you take a hard look at how you're using your technology. Are you happy with how much you're using it? Does it make you feel good most of the time? Or bad?

How would it feel to use it less? To get rid of some apps, or at least to turn off notifications on them? To set aside certain hours where you unplug? It might give your brain and your pain a chance to relax. Brett's brunch can wait.

Facing Uncertainty

In her book, *Bossypants*, Tina Fey talks about struggling with a major life decision as she approached the age of forty. Should she have a second child or should she continue focusing on her career? She felt that she needed to choose between the two options, since, as she put it, "science shows that fertility and movie offers drop off steeply for women after forty."

After months of anxiety, she found herself at her doctor's office for an annual checkup. The moment her physician entered the room, Tina burst into tears.

Her doctor listened to her anxiously weigh the pros and cons of each option, then calmly told her, "Either way, everything will be fine." That's all it took. Tina's anxiety melted away.

The feeling of uncertainty can be difficult to bear. Often we put pressure on ourselves when we're faced with the unknown:

"Should I go to UCLA, or should I go to USC?"

"Should I get a job, or should I go to grad school?"

"Should I order pizza, or should I get a salad?"

Sometimes we get so worked up about a decision that it feels like one outcome will be great and the other will be a total disaster. That kind of extreme thinking is sure to activate our danger signals. I've seen this pattern in many of my patients. They agonize over a choice. They convince themselves that it's very high stakes, which keeps their brains on high alert and exacerbates their pain.

During these times, the single best thing you can say to comfort yourself is this:

"It's going to be okay either way."

Now, does this mean that one outcome isn't preferable to another? Of course not. There's often going to be one outcome that's more desirable. But there's a difference between telling yourself, "One outcome is great and the other is a disaster," and "Both outcomes are fine, though one might be better." One is terrifying while the other one is reassuring.

Remember safety reappraisal? It's the part of somatic tracking where you send yourself messages of safety. "It's going to be okay either way" is a type of safety reappraisal that can be really effective in the face of uncertainty. It comforts your brain on a fundamental level, letting it know that you're not in danger.

Of course, 1 percent of the time, it really isn't going to be okay either way. For example, if you're told that you have a tumor, and you'll find out in three days whether it's malignant or benign, one outcome truly isn't okay. In these cases, all you can do is use whatever coping mechanisms you have to get through that waiting period, and hope for a positive outcome.

But 99 percent of the time, it really is going to be okay either way. And when you find yourself worrying about a particular outcome or agonizing over a decision, giving yourself that message can go a long way toward reducing your anxiety and helping you feel safe.

By the way, Tina Fey ended up having a second child *and* continued making movies into her forties. Which goes to show you that not only do most of the things you worry about never actually happen, but often when you stop worrying, you allow your life to unfold in ways you never could have imagined.

Patient Perspective

I used to hate texting. It sounds crazy, but I never knew what to say. If a friend asked me to hang out, I would worry that if I just wrote back, "Sure," they might think I didn't actually want to do it. But if I texted, "Definitely," maybe I'd seem too eager.

I did this with everything. I made the stakes way higher than they needed to be. When I wrote an email, should I end with "Thanks" or "Thank you"? When I went shopping, which shirt should I buy? But the worst was trying to fall asleep at night. I would lie there worrying, "If I don't fall asleep in the next ten minutes, I'm going to be exhausted tomorrow. And when I'm tired, my pain is worse."

Now I know the real thing that was making my pain worse was turning everything into a life-or-death situation. I would always go to the worst-case scenario. It was overwhelming.

Things started to turn around when I began letting myself off the hook. If I started to freak out about something minor, I would take a few deep breaths and tell myself, "It's going to be fine." If I buy a shirt and later I realize it's ugly, that's fine. I just don't have to wear it. If I don't get enough sleep, that's okay. I'll just be a little tired the next day.

Sometimes I'll still stress out in these situations—it's kind of like an automatic response. But after a few seconds, I'm like, "What am I doing?" And I'll talk myself down. In the old days, it would have been hours of anxiety—now it's two seconds.

It's funny because my girlfriend is a lot like how I used to be. She gets stressed out really easily. Because I'm such an expert in this area, it's obvious to me that she's worrying over nothing. But I've learned that it doesn't help when I point it out!

—MATTHEW

Feeling Trapped

In fall 2006, I flew to New York to attend a conference. I was looking forward to the trip. I remember feeling excited as I settled into the window seat with a handful of magazines. I had made great strides with my back pain and was ready for the flight. Or so I thought.

Fifteen minutes after sitting down, my back started hurting. I shifted around for a bit, but the pain was getting worse and worse. I knew there was only one way to get any relief: I needed to stand up and stretch my back. But when I looked over, to my horror, the guy in the middle seat was sleeping. They had just finished the safety demonstration—how was he already asleep? I was trapped.

My back was hurting already, and feeling trapped put my brain on high alert, which made the pain worse. I tried different positions. I tried sitting on my jacket. I tried using my magazines for lumbar support. Nothing helped. The rest of the flight was agony.

Most chronic pain sufferers have experienced the frustration of feeling trapped by their symptoms. It's something I see a lot in my patients that contributes to an overall sense of high alert, which makes their pain worse.

When I described the Process, I told you to use avoidance behaviors when your pain level is high. So try not to put yourself in situations where you can't practice your avoidance behaviors. Feeling trapped interferes with the Process and injects extra danger into your brain.

I made it through my flight. And I'm not going to lie, it was rough. The guy next to me woke up right before landing. He looked happy and refreshed. Part of me wanted to stuff him into the overhead compartment, but I didn't. However, I did learn a valuable lesson about feeling trapped.

The first thing I did when I landed was change my seat on the return flight so that I was sitting on the aisle. It made all the difference in the world. I could stand up, stretch, or walk to the bathroom whenever I wanted. In the end, I needed to get out of my seat only a couple of times, but knowing that I could helped me feel calm and safe.

I once had a patient with chronic dry mouth. Whenever he was stuck somewhere without easy access to a drink, he felt trapped. His anxiety would shoot through the roof and make his symptoms worse. He started carrying a bottle of water with him wherever he went. Sometimes it was inconvenient, but it made him feel safe and in control.

Another patient had joint pain and felt trapped in social situations where he had to stand for long periods of time. He and his wife had always loved going to cocktail parties with their friends, but now he started to fear them. It was hard to focus on conversations with his friends because he was panicking on the inside. "How much longer are we going to stay? How much worse is my pain going to get?" Together, we made a plan to keep him from feeling trapped. He and his wife started taking separate cars so that if he felt overwhelmed, he could go home early and not feel guilty for dragging her away. And he practiced telling his friends, "Hey, I'm really enjoying this conversation, but do you mind if we sit down? My knees are killing me." They were happy to oblige, and he was able to enjoy the parties without fear or pressure.

I encourage you to think about situations where you feel trapped by your pain. Is there a way to avoid them completely?

Is there a way to at least minimize them? The more success you have, the less fear you'll feel. Your brain will thank you.

Of course, there are going to be situations where you feel trapped and there's nothing you can do. If you're sitting in the front row of a wedding, you're not going to get up in the middle of the ceremony. No matter how much your back hurts. No matter how long the event is dragging on. Your heart may fill with fear, and your brain may go on high alert as yet another family member delivers yet another reading on the meaning of love. But let's face it, you're not going anywhere.

In situations like this, we have to rely on our old friend safety reappraisal. If we can't avoid the pain, we can at least send ourselves messages of safety: "My back hurts. I feel trapped. But it's going to be okay. This is a temporary situation. Soon the ceremony will end. The groom will kiss the bride, and I will kiss this chair goodbye and never sit in it again. I won't be trapped anymore. For the rest of the wedding I'll be free to stand up whenever I want. Cocktail hour ... dinner ... cake ... Especially cake. I'm going to eat all the cake, and I'm going to do it standing up."

CHANGING HIGH-ALERT BEHAVIORS

I started this chapter by talking about Rachel, my patient who was on high alert all the time without even realizing it. She's not alone. I've seen this pattern in my patients, my friends, and even myself. Because it's so common, it's easy to fall into the high-alert habit. It's easy to get stuck in behaviors that rev up our brains without knowing that's what we're doing. In this chapter, I've talked about the most common problem behaviors that I see: overuse of technology, struggling with uncertainty, and feeling trapped. I hope you'll think about the role these things play in your life and your pain. But please think beyond them too. Think about how you feel as you go through your day. Is there something that's causing you stress or fear or otherwise putting you on high alert? What can you do to minimize this trigger? Can you avoid it at least some of the time? Is there something you can do to reduce its impact on you? By coming up with a strategy to lower your level of high alert, you'll help your pain and your life.

That's exactly what Rachel did. Once I convinced her that the way she was feeling all day every day was not normal (or at least shouldn't be normal), she was open to making changes. The first step was to look at her high-alert behaviors to see if we could modify some of them. Here's what we found:

Rachel woke up every morning and immediately checked her phone. There were usually work texts and emails waiting for her. She hadn't brushed her teeth yet or had a single sip of coffee, and she was already on high alert. In general, mornings were frantic for Rachel. She was always running late and rushing to make it to work on time. Not exactly a calm, safe start to the day.

At work, Rachel's days were packed. She would schedule meetings back-to-back-to-back. There was no time for her to decompress.

Finally, Rachel often felt trapped at work. Not by the job itself, but by small talk. When her headaches were particularly bad, talking made them worse. And people often stopped by her office to chat. The effort of carrying on a conversation with her head throbbing was arduous, but Rachel didn't want to seem rude, so she just tried to act normal and push through the pain.

Once we'd identified Rachel's high-alert behaviors, we put together a plan to help curb them. We kept the plan very simple. Habits are hard to break, so we wanted it to be as easy as possible. Rachel agreed to the following guidelines:

- To avoid looking at her phone in the morning until she got to work;
- To set her alarm a little earlier so that she could get ready and drive to work without rushing;
- To schedule a little buffer time in between meetings whenever possible; and
- To excuse herself if she felt trapped in a conversation.

These are not drastic changes, but we thought they would be enough to improve Rachel's mental state throughout the day. It was a bit of a rocky start. The first change was the hardest for Rachel. Relying on pure willpower didn't work, because it was so easy to accidentally check her phone. Eventually, she started putting her phone in airplane mode at night and switching it back to regular mode once she got to her office.

Rachel couldn't believe how much quieter and calmer her mornings were. She was able to start each day with her brain in a safe, low-alert state. Rachel still worked hard and still had a lot of meetings. But they were spaced out better, so she had breaks in between. This allowed her to relax a bit after an intense meeting. She was still on high alert sometimes, but not all the time, and that made a big difference.

Rachel also began protecting herself when she felt trapped in a conversation. When her pain was high, she learned to politely excuse herself, and her coworkers were understanding.

Before these changes, Rachel had been struggling with the

Process. Her headaches were so frequent and so severe that she rarely had a chance to practice somatic tracking. She had been using avoidance behaviors and sending herself messages of safety, but she wasn't making progress. She felt stuck.

By tackling her high-alert habit head-on, Rachel was able to lower her overall stress level. It took time and patience, but eventually she had fewer headaches, and they were milder. She had more opportunities to use somatic tracking to get corrective experiences. She finally started gaining traction with the Process.

Your high-alert habit may be similar to Rachel's or totally different. Either way, I hope her story inspires you to make small but meaningful changes to your life to feel safer and more peaceful throughout the day.

In chapter 8, we're going to dig even deeper and look at how internal thoughts and feelings can influence chronic pain. We'll discuss strategies to reduce fear and connect with positivity in both your mind and your body.

CHAPTER 8

Getting Good at Feeling Good

There's a great parable called "The Tale of Two Wolves." It's about a conversation between a wise old man and his inquisitive young granddaughter. The girl listens eagerly as her grandfather tells her:

"There is a fight going on inside me. It is a terrible fight between two wolves.

"One is evil. He is fear, envy, regret, greed, guilt, inferiority, shame, resentment, and lies.

"The other is good. He is joy, peace, love, hope, serenity, kindness, generosity, compassion, and truth.

"The same fight is going on inside of you. This battle rages inside every person on earth."

The granddaughter's eyes get big as the old man falls silent. She finally asks, "But, Grandpa, which wolf will win?"

"The one you feed," he replies.

I love this story! It gives me chills every time. Much like the wise grandfather does, I believe everyone has both positive and negative inside them. We all succumb to fear and doubt and despair sometimes. We all delight in joy and peace and hope sometimes. But I think the balance between the two is especially important for chronic pain sufferers. And since this is a book about the neuroscience of pain, I'm not talking about mystical wolves but about the firing of neurons in your brain. ("The Tale of Two Neural Pathways" doesn't have quite the same ring to it, though.)

As you know, fear floods your brain with danger. It puts you on high alert. It makes your brain more likely to misinterpret safe sensations from your body as dangerous. Fear makes your pain worse.

Positive emotions have the opposite effect. They make you feel happy and safe. They calm your brain and put you on low alert. Positive emotions soothe your pain.

In the last chapter, I focused on behaviors that can fill your brain with a sense of danger and exacerbate your pain. This chapter is about internal thoughts and feelings that can have the same effect. I'm going to teach you how to push back against fear and connect with positivity to tip the balance away from pain and toward a safe, happy existence.

Train Your Brain

In chapter 2, I told you about the old science rule "Neurons that fire together, wire together." Different neural pathways control our thoughts, feelings, and behaviors. When we practice behaviors or have certain thoughts over and over, those neurons get "wired together." The associations between them get stronger, and they fire together more easily. Those thoughts and behaviors become more deeply rooted. On the other hand, if you don't use certain patterns for a while, the connections between those neurons get weaker. Those behaviors get rusty and those thoughts and feelings start to fade.

Pain Reprocessing Therapy is about taking control of that system. It's designed to weaken the associations that lead to pain: fear, danger, anxiety. And it reinforces the connections we want: safety, calmness, freedom.

Just as your brain can learn a new skill with practice and repetition, it can get better at certain emotional states. By reinforcing connections in your brain, you can learn to turn away from fear and gravitate toward things that feel good.

If you have negative thoughts throughout the day, you are reinforcing those associations in your brain. You are training your brain to be better and better at fear. When you stop buying into those thoughts, those neural pathways weaken. Over time, the fear fades and the negative thoughts are less frequent.

Similarly, when you cut yourself off from pleasant sensations in your body, those circuits in your brain get a little rusty. It's harder to connect with those feelings because you're out of practice. But when you lean into positive physical sensations, you'll strengthen those connections again. You'll train your brain to feel good more easily.

Don't worry, I'm not just going to tell you to "look on the bright side" or "think happy thoughts." Those sound nice but are not helpful. I'm going to give you specific techniques to reduce negative thinking and connect with positive feelings. But first, let's talk a little bit about the motivation behind these techniques.

Start with Self-Compassion

Imagine that you send your five-year-old son off to kindergarten for the first time. You pack Junior's little lunch box, zip up his backpack, and beam with pride as he walks into the classroom.

After school, you pick him up and see tears in his eyes—some second grader has been bullying him on the playground! Immediately you spring to action. You comfort Junior with a big hug and let him know he's going to be okay. You make a plan to talk to his teacher and stop the bullying. And once his tears are dry, you and Junior go out for ice cream. You both laugh as you debate the merits of mint chip versus cookies and cream.

Why do you do all this for Junior?

It's not because some parenting book told you to.

It's not because you want Junior to be well adjusted so that he can grow up, make a lot of money, and support you in your old age.

It's because you genuinely love Junior and care about how he's treated.

More than any other part of this book, this chapter is about changing the way you treat yourself. Don't make these changes just because I say so. And don't make these changes just to get out of pain. Those may be part of your motivation, but I want you to go beyond them. Make these changes because you deserve to be treated with kindness and respect. Please approach the methods in this chapter with patience and self-compassion. This is true for all of Pain Reprocessing Therapy, but it's especially true for this chapter.

Patient Perspective

When I was growing up, my parents were in a very unhappy marriage. They stayed together "for the kids." I was always the peacekeeper in my family. Always trying to be what everyone else needed me to be. It's been a lifetime of not paying attention to myself because I focused on everyone else. I always thought that was a good thing, but now I realize it's not. I look back now and I have so much sadness over how I neglected myself.

Self-compassion was a concept that I understood from an intellectual standpoint, but I wasn't sure how to get there. I took bubble baths. I ate chocolate bars. I read a thousand books on self-love. I did all those things and still felt like crap.

It wasn't until Alan had me imagine myself as a child that I was able to connect with a real feeling of caring about myself. That was the missing piece. I pictured me, about eight years old, in my brown corduroy pants. And as me the adult was looking on, I felt all this sadness because I realized all that she was carrying. When I looked at her, that's what came—this wave of wanting to reassure her and comfort her and let her know that she was okay. I didn't know really how to love myself, but this opened that door. Because she is me.

Feeling that compassion made it so much easier to be kind to myself. And that made all the difference, not just for my pain but for my whole life.

—JENNY

CATCHING YOUR FEARS

In chapter 3, I told you about three types of thoughts that trigger fear: worry, pressure, and criticism. I call these "the Big 3" because I see them again and again in my patients. They put your brain on high alert and aggravate your pain. You may tend toward one of the Big 3 or all of them.

These negative thoughts are automatic. We don't choose to have them, and we couldn't stop them if we wanted to. But that's okay. We can make the choice not to buy into them, which takes away their power. This technique is called "catching your fears" and it's a simple three-step process:

1. Notice the fear thought. This sounds easy, but it may require a little practice. These thoughts are automatic, and if you've lived with them for a long time, you may not even realize that they're negative thoughts. Pay attention to the activity of your mind to see if you can catch yourself gravitating toward fear. Once you notice a fear thought . . .

2. Don't buy into it. When we have a negative thought, our impulse is to indulge in it, to ruminate on it, to imagine a whole negative scenario playing out. Try to resist that temptation. Instead of holding on to the thought, just let it go.

3. Send yourself a message of safety. We want to replace the fear thought with a quick dose of positivity.

Every time you notice a negative thought, refuse to buy into it, and send yourself a message of safety, you are lowering the danger level in your brain. Less danger means less pain. Studies show that when pain patients catch their fears, their pain decreases.

I think as you start monitoring your own thoughts, you'll be surprised by how often fears try to sneak in. But remember, you don't have to catch every single one. Beating yourself up for not catching every criticism is just another criticism.

Here are three examples of catching your fears in action:

Worry

Dave was a patient of mine who had a tendency to worry. He worried about work. He worried about relationships. He even worried that I would stop seeing him because he worried so much.

Not surprisingly, when I started going over the techniques of Pain Reprocessing Therapy, his mind responded in the same way:

"Is my evidence sheet long enough?"

"What if I can't find any avoidance behaviors?"

"Am I doing somatic tracking right?"

Dave's worrying had become habitual. And each time he had one of these thoughts, he'd buy into it hook, line, and sinker—he'd dwell on it, he'd grapple with it, he'd think about possible consequences.

I helped Dave see what his mind was doing: that it had an infinite supply of worries ready to go at a moment's notice.

"What if I'm not able to catch them?" he asked.

"There's another one right there," I said. "See how sneaky they are?"

He started to see that his tendency to worry was just a habit. When he saw one come up, he'd simply laugh and think, "There you go again, brain." He'd let himself know that he was safe, and he'd feel proud that he was treating himself nicely.

Pressure

Dahlia was a new patient who wanted help with her neck pain. In our first session, she told me that she was getting married soon.

> **Dahlia:** So I need to be completely out of pain in six weeks, because I want the wedding to be perfect.
>
> **Me:** "Perfect" is a dangerous word because it leads to a lot of pressure. From what you've told me, you and your fiancé are deeply in love.
>
> **Dahlia:** That's true. We're crazy about each other.
>
> **Me:** And your friends and family are coming from all over the country.
>
> **Dahlia:** It's going to be everybody I love all gathered in one place, which is wonderful!
>
> **Me:** That sounds pretty amazing. Instead of putting so much pressure on yourself, do you think you could just focus on enjoying the day?
>
> **Dahlia:** Yeah, that makes sense . . . But I think the best way to enjoy the day will be if it's perfect.

Eventually, I convinced Dahlia that all this pressure was making her pain (and probably her wedding) worse. The underlying message behind all pressure thoughts is "I need to do this or else!" "Or else" is the kind of thing that fills your brain with danger. We want to replace it with messages of safety that convey that everything is going to be okay.

Dahlia started catching her pressure thoughts and telling herself, "No matter what happens, my wedding is going to be great." And it was.

It wasn't perfect. The hairdresser showed up an hour late. One of the bridesmaids wore the wrong color dress (who knew there were different shades of burgundy?). And Dahlia's neck hurt a little right before the ceremony. But Dahlia was okay with it. By taking the pressure off, she was able to enjoy her wedding, imperfections and all.

Criticism

My patient Maggie is an actor who struggled with self-criticism. After an audition, her mind would always be filled with negative thoughts: "I didn't access enough emotion." "I should have prepared more." "Why on earth did I do an old-timey accent?"

But one day, Maggie had what every actor dreams of: the audition where everything clicks. She fully embodied the character. All her creative decisions were spot-on. The casting people ate it up.

Maggie nailed it. There was absolutely nothing to critique about her performance. Then as she was driving home, a thought popped into her head: "Why did I say goodbye so weird when I left?" Which shows just how relentless critical thoughts can be.

All self-criticism basically comes down to the same idea: "There's something wrong with me." So we want to combat criticism with a message of safety that says, "There's nothing wrong with me. I'm okay the way I am."

Maggie worked on catching her fears. With practice, she got good at noticing critical thoughts, not buying into them, and telling herself, "No matter how that performance went, I know I'm a good actor. I'm okay the way I am."

Over time, Maggie's self-criticism decreased. Having fewer

critical thoughts reduced her fear, helped her pain, and made driving home after an audition a lot more pleasant (no matter which accent she did).

Building Belief (One Bug at a Time)

A common question I get from patients is "What if I don't even believe my own messages of safety?" That's completely normal. The fact that you're having negative thoughts shows that there's fear. Which means that sometimes it'll be hard to believe that everything will be okay. That's fine. Sometimes the doing comes first and the believing comes later. That's a lesson I learned from a bunch of insects.

When I was twenty, I read a book about compassion. The author had a seemingly unlimited supply of empathy for all living creatures. He said that he didn't even kill a bug when he saw one in his house. Instead, he would carefully capture it and release it outside.

The author was very convincing. With thirty seconds of effort, you can save a life! he said. I decided to give it a try. Instead of swatting flies, I carefully shooed them out of my apartment. Instead of smushing spiders, I scooped them up with a cup and a piece of paper and relocated them to the bush outside my front door.

I was treating these bugs with kindness and mercy, but the truth is that I didn't care about them at all. I was just doing it because of the book. In fact, I resented them a little because humanely catching a spider with all eight legs intact is a lot of work.

But after a few weeks, something surprising happened. A friend was hanging out at my place when he spotted a daddy longlegs in the corner and went to step on it. It was like a scene out of a movie. Everything started moving in slow motion. I screamed, "Nooooo!" and rushed toward my friend. I stopped him just in time. As I lovingly released Mr. Longlegs into the wild, I realized that by acting like I cared about these little critters, I had actually started caring about them.

Remember: "Neurons that fire together, wire together." You may not totally believe the messages of safety you give yourself, but the more you say them, the more your brain will absorb them. After all, if I can learn to feel compassion for a mosquito, you can learn to feel compassion for yourself.

From Mind to Body

Catching your fears is a great way to shift the balance in your brain away from danger and toward safety. Every time you refuse to buy into a fear thought, you take away a little negativity. And every time you send yourself a message of safety, you add a little positivity. Over time, your automatic fear thoughts will become less automatic. And your brain will gradually learn to gravitate toward positive thoughts. The end result is a calmer, safer brain.

We want to do the same thing with physical sensations. If you have chronic pain, your brain is good at experiencing negative feelings in your body. Too good. We want to help your brain unlearn those painful sensations. You're already doing that with somatic tracking.

But just like with catching your fears, there's another piece to the puzzle. It's also helpful to train your brain to seek out things that feel good. We want to strengthen the neural pathways for positive feelings. One of the best ways to do that is to connect with sensations in your body that feel nice.

But if you have chronic pain, that can be particularly challenging. It can be hard for us to explore the positive sensations in our bodies because our fear keeps getting in the way. My friend Jane has a similar problem with a different kind of fear.

SCANNING FOR THREATS

Jane is deathly afraid of dogs. She hates admitting it, because people always respond the same way: "What? But dogs are so cuuuute!" (I said this exact sentence when Jane told me.) Jane never knows what to say to that, because to her, dogs aren't cute—they're terrifying.

Jane has a good reason for her fear. Like many people with cynophobia, Jane had a traumatic experience with a dog in her childhood. Jane was at a friend's house for a playdate when the friend's dog—a high-strung cocker spaniel—freaked out, chased Jane around the yard, and bit her on the leg.

You've probably heard the expression "Once bitten, twice shy." Well Jane is once bitten, a hundred times shy. She experiences a huge amount of anxiety whenever she's around a dog. Big dogs are worse than small dogs, but pretty much any canine will trigger Jane's fear. Even this guy:

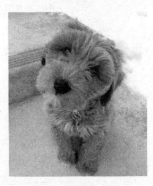

"I would never hurt you, Jane."

When she does find herself around a dog, Jane is completely on edge. All her attention is focused on being vigilant. "Is it going to jump on me?" "Is it going to chase me?" "Is it going to bite me?"

I understand Jane's fear, but it makes me sad. Because of one traumatic event, she's missing out on so many wonderful dog experiences: playing fetch, going for walks, scratching their bellies until they do that crazy leg-kicking thing. (What's up with that thing?) Dogs are pretty much happiness in animal form, but Jane's anxiety keeps her from enjoying it. It's a shame, but many chronic pain sufferers experience something similar with our own bodies. Just as Jane was traumatized by that cocker spaniel, we've been traumatized by our pain. Just as Jane is scared of all dogs, we can start to see our bodies as nothing but a source of pain and fear.

When Jane is around a dog, she's constantly scanning for threats. But when you have chronic pain, the threats aren't sitting and panting a few feet away—they're inside you. Which is why many pain sufferers continually scan their own bodies for problems. This is known as "hypervigilance."

It's a form of internal high alert where you can become paranoid of every little twinge or sensation in your body. "Is something wrong?" "Is that pain?" "Is that some kind of pre-pain where it's not quite pain, but maybe it will turn into pain later?!"

When you're hypervigilant, you get so caught up in scanning your body for negative sensations that you cut yourself off from the positive ones. But connecting with pleasant feelings is a great way to make your brain feel safe and start building a healthier relationship with your body.

EMBRACING POSITIVE SENSATIONS

When I first started having symptoms, I existed in one of two states: I was either in pain or I was waiting for the pain to strike. Every sensation was a potential threat. If I felt nothing, I'd brace for that first little twinge. If I had a hint of pain, I'd lock in on it and wait for it to get worse. It's like my own body had become my enemy.

As I began using somatic tracking, catching my fears, and giving myself messages of safety, my pain gradually decreased. I was feeling a lot better, but I still didn't trust my body. I saw it as a source of danger.

I wanted to change that. I didn't just want to feel less bad; I wanted to feel good.

I remember taking a walk around the block and opening myself up to positive sensations: the sun on my skin, the breeze against my face, even the feeling of my breath rising and falling. I couldn't believe how easy it was! I'd taken a million walks before, where had these sensations been? Even my other senses were getting in on the action. The smell of freshly cut grass, the birds chirping in the background, everything just seemed . . . nice.

I decided to make a practice of it. Throughout the day, I'd bring my attention to sensations that felt good. Sometimes they were there, and sometimes they weren't. I realized that you couldn't force feeling good; you could only open yourself up to it. But the more I practiced, the more my attention went there automatically. After years of treating my body as the enemy, I began seeing it as an ally.

Embracing positive sensations helps your brain feel safe.

And there are so many of them out there! When we make an effort to connect with these feelings, we can learn to trust our bodies again.

As you go through your day, see if you can lean in to positive sensations. You don't need to do anything extra—just take advantage of the sensations that are already there. If you're taking a hot shower, focus on the nice feeling of the water hitting your skin. If you're stretching in the morning, lean in to the pleasant tension of your muscles. If you like the feeling of your breath flowing in and out of your body, take a few moments to really enjoy it.

How often should you lean in to positive feelings? As often as you want! It's easy and it feels good. The more you practice embracing these sensations, the easier it becomes. And over time, you'll come to see your body as an ally once again.

REX'S STORY

I thought it would help to share a recovery story that involves the techniques we covered in this chapter. So here's the case of a patient named Rex, who overcame a lawn mower, an eight-mile run, and decades of pressure to heal his pain.

One day in the summer of 2000, Rex was mowing his lawn when he felt a tweak in his back. By the next morning, he was in so much pain that he couldn't get out of bed. He rested it, he iced it, but it didn't improve. For the next eighteen years, through an endless string of doctors' appointments, physical therapy treatments, and acupuncture sessions, Rex's pain persisted. He cursed that lawn mower more times than he could count.

When I first met Rex, he was skeptical that his pain was neuroplastic. He'd always believed that the lawn mower incident caused some sort of structural damage to his back. Whenever he had a flare-up, he would tell himself, "I must have lifted something heavy." Or, "I overdid it." He always came up with some kind of physical reason after the fact.

As Rex and I started gathering evidence and noticing exceptions, he saw that his physical explanations didn't always fit. He came to accept that his pain was neuroplastic and finally stopped blaming his innocent lawn mower. But soon we encountered another barrier: Rex had a hard time with self-compassion.

When Rex was ten years old, he would lie in bed and imagine opening a store someday. And then he would think, "What if nobody came and bought anything?" He hadn't even graduated elementary school and he was already anticipating bankruptcy.

As an adult, Rex is a successful businessman. But according to him, he had that same "gripping fear of failure" that he had as a child. And because of it, he put enormous pressure on himself:

"I have to succeed."

"I can't let these investors down."

"I've got to take care of my family."

Not surprisingly, this pressure carried over to our sessions. He didn't want to fail treatment. He didn't want to fail me. And he put a lot of pressure on himself to beat the pain.

We had a conversation during one of our early sessions that really drove this point home:

Rex: I went for a run yesterday, and almost immediately it was like I'd blown out my whole spine. My back was spasming, and I was in a lot of pain.

Me: I'm so sorry to hear that! What did you do?

Rex: I finished the run.

He put so much pressure on himself that he didn't even want to fail a leisurely run.

I started working with Rex on self-compassion. We talked about that ten-year-old kid who used to lie in bed and terrify himself about the future. He was sad about how much pressure that kid felt, and that helped him see that he was still treating himself that same way.

Rex began catching his fears. When his mind went to that familiar place of pressure or worry, he intervened. He didn't want to do that to himself anymore.

It took time, but Rex began to change. Success still mattered to him, but taking care of himself mattered more. I taught him somatic tracking, the rules of the Process, and to embrace positive sensations. He used them all, but he took care to apply them without pressure or urgency.

Rex eventually overcame his symptoms, but the thing he was most proud of was that he prioritized feeling good over being perfect.

Like Rex, you might have the tendency to treat yourself in a negative way. You may have been doing so without even realizing it. But it matters how you're treated. And by fostering self-compassion, catching your fears, and embracing positive feelings, you're taking the steps you need to help your brain feel safe.

In chapter 9, we'll discuss relapses, resilience, and taking ownership of your recovery. I'll tell you what to expect from a relapse, how to bounce back from one, and, best of all, how to prevent them in the first place.

CHAPTER 9

Relapses, Resilience, and Recovery

In chapter 1, I told you about Casey. He's the baseball-playing high school student that I treated on *The Doctors*. Using Pain Reprocessing Therapy, Casey was able to eliminate his crippling abdominal pain. Since I'd last seen him, Casey had graduated from high school and enrolled at a local community college. He also worked part-time and played in an adult softball league with his dad. (How great is that?) His pain had been gone for two years, and Casey was living his best life.

Until, out of the blue, I got this text message from his mom: "Hi Alan, this is Dianna. Casey is being taken to the hospital by ambulance with pain in the same place as before."

His pain was back, and it was bad enough to call an ambulance. Casey was having a relapse.

I called Casey's mom and arranged to see him as soon as possible. Casey was in shock. He thought he was done with the pain for good. The first thing I did was reassure Casey that relapses happen. He beat the pain once before and he could do it again.

We talked about why the pain may have returned. In my experience, relapses can happen for a few reasons. Sometimes a stressful event puts the brain on high alert and triggers pain. Sometimes patients fall back into old habits like high-alert behaviors or negative thinking. Or sometimes patients will get injured or think they got injured. If they become preoccupied with the injury, they get pulled back into the pain-fear cycle.

Casey thought that he might have pulled a muscle playing catch with his dad a couple of weeks before. (I love this family.) I think it's interesting that Casey's first thought was that it was a physical injury. Even though the game of catch was two weeks prior to his relapse. Even though he went on national television and cured his pain with a mind-body approach. Even though his pain came back in exactly the same spot where he had neuroplastic pain before. Despite all that, Casey's brain immediately jumped to a structural cause for his pain.

I'm not knocking Casey. I do the exact same thing. I think and talk about neuroplastic pain all day, every day. And yet every time I have a new symptom, my first instinct is "Maybe I injured something!" It shows how tempting it is to believe that pain must be coming from the body. The evidence sheets that I described in chapter 4 help with relapses too.

I told Casey that I was skeptical that his game of catch was the cause, but that even if he had strained a muscle, it would heal and his pain would go away. I had a different theory about the return of Casey's pain. He told me that he'd recently gotten a promotion at work and that his new role had a lot more responsibility and stress. I thought this new stress had triggered his relapse.

Regardless of the exact cause, we needed to get Casey back to his pain-free life. After all, he and his dad had softball games to win!

Three Stages and You're Out

I've noticed that when my patients relapse, they always go through the same three stages.

STAGE 1: PANIC

Getting out of chronic pain is an amazing feeling. It's like you're finally free. A relapse feels like the exact opposite. Like you're back to square one. You can't believe this nightmare that you thought was gone is back. It's demoralizing.

When Casey walked into my office for the first time in two years, I could see Stage 1 written all over his face. He didn't even think a relapse was possible. He had completely moved on. So when the pain came back, he was blindsided. The poor guy was terrified.

We decided to try a somatic tracking exercise. Casey did his best to relax. He closed his eyes and brought his attention to the pain in his stomach. He tried to observe it with lightness and curiosity.

It didn't work at all. There was no lightness. There was no curiosity.

It was clear that Casey was just too scared. In this state, he couldn't have watched a butterfly with lightness and curiosity, much less the source of his fear. There's no way he could get a corrective experience. But that's okay. As we know from the Process, timing is important. I told Casey that we'd try again later and that in the meantime he should focus on sending himself messages of safety.

Casey was in Stage 1 for his first two sessions with me. But he stayed focused on communicating safety. "It's going to be all right. I'm just in shock right now. But I overcame it once before, and I will do it again. I'm safe." After a week or two, his brain absorbed these messages and lowered its alert level. When Casey came in for our third session, he had moved on to . . .

STAGE 2: FORCING IT

In the movie *Groundhog Day*, Bill Murray is stuck in a time loop, living the same day over and over. In the middle of the movie, he goes on an amazing date with Andie MacDowell. Their time together is authentic and surprising. There's even a spontaneous snowball fight. The laughter and chemistry are off the charts.

The next day (which is really the same day), Bill Murray tries to re-create the date. But this time it's not authentic or surprising. He's saying the same romantic things he said last time. He's throwing the same snowballs. But just as a means to an end. Andie MacDowell can feel that something is off. It's nothing like the first date; the magic just isn't there.

Stage 2 of a pain relapse is exactly like that second date. In Stage 2, patients have overcome the panic of Stage 1. They are doing all the right things, but with the wrong mindset. They're doing somatic tracking and sending themselves messages of safety, but instead of self-compassion and lightness, they're doing it with an undercurrent of desperation and pressure. So, naturally, none of it works.

When Casey came in for his third session, he was deep in Stage 2. He was frustrated. "It's not working this time! I forgot how to do it." I told him about *Groundhog Day*. I told him that he was trying to force something a second time that happened organically the first time.

We went over the somatic tracking guidelines that I told you about in chapter 5: turning down the intensity and being outcome independent. More than anything else we talked about the importance of making his brain feel safe, not just with the techniques but also with the spirit behind the techniques. He took a deep breath and promised to try. Finally, I told him, "Look on the bright side—there's only one stage left!"

STAGE 3: "OH YEAH, THIS IS HOW IT WORKS!"

After the terror of Stage 1 and the frustration of Stage 2, Stage 3 is when everything clicks again. Patients are now doing the right things and with the right energy. And it works! Stage 3 is when the relapse goes away and all's right with the universe again.

I never got to see Casey in Stage 3. He had promised to turn down the intensity and approach his recovery from a place of peace and positivity. And he was true to his word. The day before our fourth appointment, I got a text from Casey: "I don't think we need to meet tomorrow 'cause I'm doing really good." Once he had the right mindset, he was able to use somatic tracking to remind his brain how to properly process the signals from his body. And his pain went away.

This is the key to Stage 3. After a relapse, you get rid of the pain the same way you did before. Because there's only one path out of neuroplastic pain. You overcome your symptoms when your brain learns that the pain is a false alarm—that the sensations it's been misinterpreting are actually safe.

I had a huge grin on my face as I texted Casey back, "No problem!"

Whenever one of my patients has a relapse, I tell them about the three stages. And then we have this conversation:

> **Patient:** Now that I know about the three stages, can I go straight to Stage 3?
>
> **Me:** No.

I wish my patients could skip the first two stages, but everyone has to go through them. Even though I tell them exactly what's going to happen, it still happens. The pain coming back is just such a big shock. It's impossible not to freak out in Stage 1. It's impossible not to feel desperate in Stage 2. It takes time to get past that shock. For Casey it took a few weeks. For some patients it takes only a few days or, for a lucky few, just a couple of hours.

I hope you don't have a relapse, but if you do, it helps to know how it's going to play out. And it's especially helpful to know that it has a happy ending. No matter how crushing it seems in the moment, you can bounce back. That's a lesson I learned long before I ever had pain.

Road Trip, Rejection, and Resilience

My senior year of college at UCLA, I was majoring in economics and interviewing for jobs at management consulting firms. There was just one problem—I hated economics, and I didn't want to be a management consultant.

My real dream was to be on *Saturday Night Live*. Throughout college, I wrote and performed comedy songs (think Adam

Sandler meets Weird Al Yankovic). It was the thing I enjoyed most.

One day, after a particularly boring econ lecture, I'd had enough. I dropped all my classes, hopped in my car, and drove to New York City. The entire trip there, I rehearsed the speech I was going to give to *SNL* producer Lorne Michaels:

"Mr. Michaels, you give me three minutes onstage, and I'll bring the house down like you've never seen before." (My level of confidence was inversely proportional to my grasp on reality.)

When I got to 30 Rockefeller Plaza, I grabbed my guitar and headed inside to meet my destiny. There was a security guard at the elevator.

Guard: What floor, please?

Me: *Saturday Night Live* floor!

Guard: Where's your pass?

Me: My pass?

I didn't make it past the elevator. Apparently you can't just wander in off the street and give speeches to Lorne Michaels.

As I walked back to my car, I was crushed. My dream was dead.

It was a very long drive back to Los Angeles, but somewhere between Ohio and Oklahoma I had an epiphany. I wasn't on *Saturday Night Live*, but that didn't mean I had to be a management consultant. I truly loved comedy, and I was going to find a way to do it for a living. In other words, I bounced back.

After I re-enrolled at UCLA and finished my degree, I started pursuing comedy. I was thrilled to be following my dream, but my lessons in resilience were just beginning. I started performing at open-mic nights. Sometimes the crowd loved me. Other times they tolerated me. Once, there were three people in the audience, and only one of them laughed. And it was a pity laugh. But I kept going.

Each time I bounced back from a setback, it deepened my faith in my own resilience. I wrote new songs and tested them out on different crowds. When they didn't work, I rewrote them. Over time, my songs got funnier, and I improved as a performer.

I moved from open-mic nights to clubs to festivals. I started booking gigs at colleges, and soon I was touring all around the country, performing such classics as "Roommate from Hell," "Three Finals in One Day," and the ever-controversial "Sorority Song." I had done it. I was making a living with comedy, and it was all because when the going got tough, I kept going.

Ultimately, I decided to pursue a different dream, but the resilience that I developed in my comedy days has served me well in everything I've done since. And nowhere was it more important than in my struggles with pain.

MORE RESILIENCE, LESS FEAR

Resilience is helpful for every part of the pain recovery process: relapses, extinction bursts, and especially setbacks. In chapter 6, I encouraged you to minimize setbacks as part of the Process. But they're still going to happen.

As bad as setbacks feel, they actually give us opportunities to build resilience. And building resilience is what leads to a reduction of fear. For example, the first few times I bombed onstage, I was devastated. I was sweating from pores I didn't even know I had. But I gave myself little pep talks:

"It's just one night."

"I'm going to get better with practice."

"Even Jay Leno was terrible when he first started."

These messages of safety helped me bounce back. After a few months of being onstage, the prospect of bombing was a lot less scary because I'd recovered from it so many times before.

And the same is true with pain. When you have a setback, it's very easy to get sucked into hopelessness and despair. But giving yourself messages of safety helps protect you from those feelings. You bounce back. And the more you recover, the greater your belief in your ability to recover.

Don't worry if you don't think of yourself as a resilient person. The truth about resilience is that it's a learned behavior. If you gravitate toward hopelessness, it's not because you're hopeless, but because your brain has done it so many times before. If your mind naturally goes to despair, it's not because your situation is dire, but because you have developed strong neural pathways for despair.

Science has shown that you can become more resilient through practice. The techniques in this book—practicing self-compassion, catching your fears, sending messages of safety—will help you build up your ability to bounce back from adversity.

Patient Perspective

I'm an active guy. I define myself as an athlete. That was the hardest thing about my hip pain. I couldn't do the physical activities I liked. I wasn't able to be me.

When I had good days, I was able to feel hopeful. But whenever my pain would ramp up, it was devastating. I would think, "I'll never be able to ski again. I'll never be able to work out again. I'll never be able to run around with my kids again." I grappled and worried and went over obsessively in my mind all sorts of catastrophic outcomes.

I knew that responding to the pain with all this despair and fear was keeping the pain alive. I needed to break this habit, but the pull to hopelessness and catastrophe was so strong. It was very, very hard not to go down that path. I had to try a bunch of different things. If I had to put my finger on it and say what got me out of this, it was thinking about that Robert Frost poem and how he takes the road "less traveled."

If I felt the pain come on, I'd think, "Okay, right–take the road less traveled, don't react the way you normally do. This is just your brain misinterpreting signals. You know you've been through this before. It's not permanent."

My focus had totally changed. I used to obsess and worry about whether my hip was going to start hurting, but that stopped mattering as much. The important thing was how I reacted when the pain did come on.

Sometimes the gravitational pull was too strong and I couldn't help feeling despair. But more and more, I was able to take the road less traveled. The pain lost its power over me and eventually faded.

> My life is easier now because I'm not constantly being hyper-vigilant over whether I'm going to have an unpleasant sensation. Even today at the gym, I was rowing and I felt something in my hip. At first there was that feeling of fear, but then I just laughed it off and went about my day.
>
> —KYLE

The Great Motivator

If you have a relapse, resilience will help you work your way through the three stages and back out of pain. But even better than bouncing back is not having a relapse in the first place. The key to staying out of pain is the same as the key to getting out of pain: you want to make your brain feel safe. Everything we've covered in this book is designed for that exact purpose.

- making evidence sheets
- practicing somatic tracking
- using avoidance behaviors
- sending messages of safety
- reducing overstimulation
- avoiding feeling trapped
- handling uncertainty
- catching your fears
- embracing positive sensations

These are all very different techniques, but they all do the same thing. They make your brain feel safe, calm your high-alert state, and turn off neuroplastic pain. Just as these techniques can get you out of pain, they can keep you out. The hard part is remembering to use them.

Pain is the great motivator. It's a constant reminder that you have a problem you need to fix. The fact that it's a loud, furious reminder is what makes it so effective. When I had chronic pain, I would do anything to make it stop. I went to endless doctors' appointments, endured painful tests, tried every treatment. If you had told me I could cure my pain by starting each morning with a root canal, I would have been in the dentist's chair at 7:00 a.m. That's how motivated I was.

Once we're out of pain, we don't have that constant reminder anymore, and it's easy to fall back into the old way of doing things. It's easy to start obsessing about a possible injury. It's easy to go back to criticizing yourself. It's easy for your phone to be the first thing you see every morning and the last thing you see every night.

So even once your pain is gone, keep taking care of yourself. Use the techniques in this book regularly to maintain a safe, pain-free brain. But keep it simple. You don't want to overwhelm yourself. We've all made those overly ambitious New Year's resolutions where we promise to work out every day, eat perfectly healthy, and cut out TV. By January 4, we're on the couch, knee-deep in french fries and binge-watching *Friends*.

If you set manageable goals, you're more likely to stick with them. Pick one or two techniques that resonate with you the most and incorporate them into your daily life. If you struggle with negative thoughts, keep catching your fears. If your phone has a tendency to put you on high alert, keep setting some limits. The important thing is to keep taking care of yourself on a consistent basis.

I reached out to a couple of former patients to see what they've been doing to maintain their recovery since they finished treatment. Here's what they had to say.

Amir told me:

> *The main thing for me is checking in with my body. It was hard to remember to check in at first, so I started using a cue. I would check in every time I got a phone call (I can get twenty-five to forty of these a day). My check-in is very quick—a deep breath or two—and I'm able to do it and still be cognizant of my surroundings and do my job.*

Imagine a bucket that's constantly filling up with water. If you dump the bucket out every time the water reaches an inch high, it'll never overflow. This is essentially Amir's relapse-prevention strategy. When he checks in with positive sensations in his body (mainly his breath), it always calms him down. By doing this throughout the day, he keeps himself from going to a high-alert place and protects himself from pain.

Of course, when you're out of pain, it can be hard to remember to engage in activities that soothe your brain. Amir uses the brilliant system of checking in every time he gets a work call. And Amir gets a lot of work calls! By using them as a built-in reminder, Amir keeps his stress level well regulated.

Carla shared:

> *Every morning I spend five minutes in bed setting my intention for the day. It helps me start my day on the right track. I even made a self-compassion recording for myself, though I don't listen to it every day.*

To be honest, I still have a little pain now and then. I don't consider myself a chronic pain person anymore, but I still have a minor flare-up occasionally. For a while I was frustrated that it wasn't totally gone (perfectionist? who, me?), but I've actually started looking at it as a little helper. If I'm running around like crazy or putting too much pressure on myself, my body tells me loud and clear. So instead of getting mad, I try to listen to it and give myself what I need.

I love the amount of self-compassion Carla has. She's making sure to take care of herself every morning. And even though she has a little residual pain, she's not putting too much pressure on herself about it. That attitude of patience and self-acceptance keeps her brain calm. I've worked with a lot of pain patients who will be 90 percent better and beat themselves up for not being at 100 percent. But you don't have to be perfect to be good enough.

Carla's pain is low enough and infrequent enough that she can thoroughly enjoy her life. And instead of resenting the fact that it's not completely gone, she looks at the pain as a helpful reminder, like a lighthouse in the night, illuminating something that she might not otherwise have seen. I can't think of a better example of giving yourself messages of safety.

Paving Your Own Path

Shelley Berman was a stand-up comedian in the 1950s and '60s. He used to tell a joke about his grandfather immigrating to America. Shelley's grandpa had heard that America was the land of opportunity, that the streets were paved with gold! But when he finally arrived in America, he learned three things:

1. The streets were not paved with gold.

2. The streets were not paved.

3. He was the guy who was going to be paving them.

Often when we look outside ourselves for salvation, we're searching in the wrong place, because we have the power to create the life we wanted all along.

When I was in chronic pain, I was desperately looking for someone who could cure me. Each new practitioner brought a fresh sense of hope, and each failed treatment brought crushing disappointment.

When I learned about neuroplastic pain, it changed my perspective. I realized it was *my* brain that was making a mistake, so only *my* brain had the power to fix it. This notion was a little scary. After all, I'd been looking to others to cure my pain for so long. But it was also empowering: I had the capacity to heal myself!

Everyone has the power to fix their own pain. Over the years, I've worked with many patients who have overcome their symptoms. But the truth is, I never healed any of them. I just gave them the tools to heal themselves. And now I've given those tools to you.

After reading this book, you understand how the brain generates pain based on signals from the body. You know that this system isn't perfect—the brain can make mistakes and give off false alarms. You've seen how fear fuels these mistakes and leads to an endless loop called the pain-fear cycle. You know that believing your body is damaged feeds into that fear and keeps the pain stuck.

You learned about the different components of somatic tracking and how they work together to turn off the false alarm. You studied the rules of the Process to know how and when to use somatic tracking for maximum effect. You went over techniques to calm your brain, catch your fears, and embrace positive feelings.

You read about how to use each tool, the science behind it, and the strategy for applying it. And now it's time to pave your own path.

The fundamentals of Pain Reprocessing Therapy are universal: Fear is the fuel for the pain. Safety is the key to breaking the pain-fear cycle. But the specifics vary. I trust you to figure out what resonates with you and heal yourself. I've given you a toolbox, but you're the one who's going to take these tools and get yourself out of pain.

I named this book *The Way Out* because I know what it feels like to be trapped by chronic pain. It screams at you, it beats you down, it steals your joy, it haunts your thoughts, and all you want more than anything in the world is a way out.

And when you've been in pain for months or years, you want that freedom to come as soon as possible. But please be patient with yourself. It takes time to form new habits; it takes practice to develop new neural pathways. But every day going forward, you can change your brain a little bit more. Each setback is an opportunity for resilience. Each twinge is a shot at a corrective experience. Each fear is a chance for a message of safety.

We may have reached the end of the book, but for you, it's just the beginning. The way out of pain starts now.

The State of Healthcare and the Opioid Crisis

In the fall of 2012, I started working with Brian, a new patient with terrible back pain. Over the next few months, he learned and applied the principles of Pain Reprocessing Therapy and eventually overcame his symptoms. But this isn't the story of Brian's recovery; this is the story of everything he went through in the twenty years before.

Brian's Story, Part I: Hope and Disappointment

It all started with a twinge.

One morning in 1992, Brian was out for a run. He loved jogging really early when everyone else was still asleep. It gave him a sense of peace. But there was nothing peaceful about his run this morning. About two miles in, he felt a twinge of pain in his lower back. He didn't think much of it at the time, but that little

twinge led to decades of doctors' appointments, medical procedures, major surgeries, and eventually an opioid addiction.

When Brian first hurt his back, he set out to identify the
cause. He's an accountant by trade, and if there's one thing he's
learned in his career, it's this: where there's a problem, there's
a solution. He got an MRI and learned that he had a bulging
disc. Three different orthopedists recommended physical therapy. So he threw himself into physical therapy like no one ever
had: three times a week, every week, for two years.

Then, 312 physical therapy sessions later, he returned to his
doctors. "I'm still in pain," he said. "What else can we try?"

The physicians recommended an epidural injection. The
epidural was done under a live X-ray so that they could inject
cortisone right into his disc. But the shot didn't help, so he got
another. And then another. All to no avail.

Brian was frustrated and desperate. The only thing left to
try was spinal fusion surgery, but his doctors were reluctant.
It's a major surgery and it's irreversible. The doctors pointed
out that Brian's main pain triggers were sitting or doing physical activity. They asked, "Can't you just avoid those things?"
But Brian was an accountant and a fitness enthusiast—his
whole life was sitting and doing physical activity!

Because Brian had exhausted all other options, his doctors
agreed to do the surgery. They removed the disc that they
thought was the problem and installed hardware to help the
vertebrae fuse together. The surgery went smoothly, and Brian
dove into his recovery. After two months of physical therapy,
he returned to work, feeling optimistic. Unfortunately, his
pain returned as well. Sitting in his office, Brian felt the familiar agony in his back. He was crushed. "It was the worst thing

in the world," he said. "Hope, then disappointment." The surgery was a complete failure.

It's heartbreaking to hear that Brian went through major surgery for nothing, but it's not surprising. Studies have compared spinal fusion for back pain with other nonsurgical treatments. They found that patients did about the same whether they had surgery or not. Except those who had surgery had a much greater risk of complications, like infection and even paralysis.

The beauty of science is that we're constantly increasing our knowledge to make better decisions. Once it was established that this surgery was ineffective, it should have fallen out of favor. But in the years following the publication of these studies, the number of fusion surgeries in the United States actually went up! How could that be? There are several reasons, among them a lack of better treatment options and increasing rates of chronic pain. But to a large degree it's because we're so attached to the idea that pain always comes from the body that we keep trying to fix the body. Even when it means ignoring the science.

Brian's Story, Part II: The Price of Pain

After his surgery, Brian was back at work and back in pain. He tried another epidural, which didn't work. He did another year of physical therapy, which didn't help. He even got a second surgery, but that only seemed to make things worse.

Meanwhile Brian's bills were piling up. He was fortunate to have health insurance, but there were still a lot of expenses. He had to cover copays and deductibles. He had to take time off work for appointments. He bought special chairs and standing desks and medical devices.

So how much did Brian spend? Given that he's a fastidious accountant, we don't have to guess. Over twenty years, Brian's pain cost him $83,417. And he has the receipts to prove it.

Pain is expensive! The total cost of chronic pain in the United States is more than $600 billion annually. That's the equivalent of buying every chronic pain sufferer in the country a new Rolex every year. But even though we're spending all this money, it's not getting people out of pain.

And that's what's so frustrating. Whether you measure it in thousands of dollars per person or billions for society as a whole, the cost of chronic pain is too high, because we're spending the money on treatments that don't work. Which is why Brian, like so many pain sufferers, was eventually told, "You will always have pain. All you can do is try to manage it."

Brian's Story, Part III: Opioids

For the next fifteen years, the pain was always there. "My whole life was run by pain," he said. "It was never-ending."

His doctors had exhausted all of their treatment options, so they sent him to pain management, which consisted entirely of prescribing opioids. He was given an opioid painkiller called Ultram (also known as tramadol) to take twice a day. He was in near constant pain, and the Ultram helped somewhat. He told me, "I was always watching the clock for the next Ultram. Sometimes after lunch I would realize it was only 2:00 p.m., but I had to wait until 3:00. People who worked with me and knew me, they could see the pain in my eyes. They felt sorry for me."

At various points during his two decades in pain, Brian took Ultram, codeine, methadone, and OxyContin—all opioids and all addictive. Once he was out of pain, Brian worked with an addiction medicine specialist to wean himself off the drugs. He said, "It was really tough to get off the opioids. It would have been almost impossible to get off them when I was in pain."

Which brings us to the opioid crisis. And it is indeed a crisis. In 2017, more than 56 million Americans were prescribed some kind of opioid painkiller. Of course, these drugs can serve a legitimate purpose: short-term pain reduction. But in the long term, patients build up a tolerance to opioids, which become less effective. Not to mention that they are addictive and dangerous. Opioid overdoses are now the leading cause of accidental death in the United States, more lethal than guns or car accidents. Opioid deaths are so common that the average American's life expectancy has actually gone down for the past three years. The last time that happened we were simultaneously fighting World War I and dealing with a global flu epidemic.

In response to the opioid crisis, the Centers for Disease Control has set new guidelines to reduce painkiller prescriptions. But this has led to a new fear: that chronic pain patients like Brian won't be able to get the opioids that help them make it through the day.

When it comes to chronic pain, opioids are a Band-Aid solution at best. They may provide some relief, but they don't treat the underlying source of the pain. However, making opioids harder to get is not a solution either. Even if we resolve the opioid crisis, which I sincerely hope we do, that does nothing to address the pain crisis. What we need is a new approach to chronic pain.

A New Way

For more than two decades, Brian suffered through unnecessary surgeries, ineffective injections, and addictive painkillers. But I want to be clear that Brian's doctors are not the villains of this story. During his twenty-year odyssey, Brian dealt with dozens of medical practitioners, and for the most part, they were caring and cautious. They did their best to treat Brian's pain with the tools they had. The problem is that they were using the wrong tools.

To become a doctor, students must go to medical school for four to six years (depending on the country). Medical students spend thousands of hours learning everything from anatomy to genetics. So how much of the medical school curriculum is devoted to pain? In the United States, it's eleven hours. Not eleven hours per class. Not even eleven hours per year. Eleven hours of pain content in the entire four-year curriculum. The rest of the world doesn't fare much better. In Europe, it's twelve hours. In the U.K., it's thirteen. Canada, Australia, and New Zealand are on the high end, with twenty hours dedicated to pain.

Eleven hours?! Twenty hours?! Of all the stories, studies, and statistics that I've presented in this book, this is the most mind-boggling. In school, I spent at least thirty hours learning the periodic table of the elements. I have used that knowledge exactly zero times. And yet future doctors are spending less time than that studying something that afflicts more than a billion people worldwide!

This lack of pain education reflects the old way of thinking: That pain is just a symptom. That pain is always caused by some kind of injury, damage, or disease in the body. But that's a twentieth-century idea. Thanks to cutting-edge fMRI studies, we now know that neuroplastic pain is a disease unto itself. Neuroplastic pain is a fundamentally different kind of pain. It's perpetuated by the brain, and it needs to be treated in the brain.

In the last twenty years, our understanding of chronic pain has exploded, and yet my team and I see patients every day who are still being given the same ineffective treatments as Brian was. And naturally, they stay in pain. Everything Brian went through may sound extreme, but the depressing truth is that his experience is common. The patients in the Boulder Back Pain Study had been in pain for an average of eleven years. And most of them have their own laundry lists of unsuccessful medical treatments.

We can do better. We need to do better. I'm not talking about small, incremental improvements. What we need is a major paradigm shift in how we view and treat chronic pain. Our understanding of pain has evolved, and it's time for our healthcare system to follow suit. Modern medicine needs to embrace the new findings in the neuroscience of pain. Doctors need to replace old, inadequate treatments with new evidence-based therapies. We must make pain education a priority and teach the doctors of tomorrow that pain is much more than a simple reaction to the body.

We've done the hard part. Scientists all over the world have contributed to a completely new understanding of what chronic pain is and how it works. Now we need to use that knowledge to help the millions of Brians out there who are still suffering.

Throughout human history, we have used reason and science to solve seemingly impossible problems. To help us live better and longer. We've conquered diseases that once plagued millions: scurvy, polio, smallpox. It's time to add chronic pain to that list.

appendix

How to Determine If You Have Neuroplastic Pain

There's one question I get more than any other. Pain sufferers will describe their symptoms to me and then ask, "Is this neuroplastic?" My answer is always the same: "It *could* be."

The brain is capable of generating any physical sensation in any part of the body: Pain in your back, your neck, your eyes, your teeth. Muscle pain, nerve pain, sharp pain, dull pain. Tightness, tingling, burning, numbness. If you're experiencing an unpleasant sensation anywhere in your body, it is absolutely possible that it's neuroplastic.

But how do you know if it is?

As I mention in chapter 2, most chronic pain is neuroplastic. That said, chronic pain conditions can be caused by physical problems in the body, such as tumors, infections, fractures, and autoimmune disorders.

Because all pain *feels* like it's coming from the body, it can be difficult to distinguish between pain that's physically caused and pain that's neuroplastic. Luckily, there are certain signs you can look for that point to neuroplastic pain. Here is a list of guidelines that can help you make this determination.

Pain Originated During Time of Stress

About half the patients I've worked with had their pain first appear during a particularly stressful time. Maybe their job was really intense, or they just had a new baby. Maybe they were under a lot of financial stress or had recently lost a loved one. As I discuss in chapter 3, stress puts the brain on high alert and can trigger pain. So if your symptoms started during a stressful time, that points to neuroplastic pain.

Pain Originated Without Injury

If your pain first came on without any preceding injury, that's a sign that it's neuroplastic.

But what if you did injure yourself? I've seen a number of patients whose neuroplastic pain started with an injury. One patient pulled his hamstring during a soccer game. Another hurt her neck in a car accident. A third slipped on some ice and sprained his wrist.

At first their pain was appropriate—it was due to actual tissue damage in their bodies. But after their injuries healed, their pain persisted. It became neuroplastic. So even if your pain started with an injury, if you're past the normal course of healing, it's likely neuroplastic.

Symptoms Are Inconsistent

Often patients with neuroplastic pain have inconsistent symptoms. I had one patient who liked to take walks around the block, but sometimes he would have pain and sometimes he wouldn't. I had another patient who always had pain when she drove, but sometimes it was a 2 out of 10 and sometimes it was a 7 out of 10. A third patient had pretty bad pain Monday through Friday, but on the weekend it was hardly noticeable.

This kind of inconsistency is a big sign that your pain is neuroplastic. Structurally caused pain generally doesn't have this type of variation.

Large Number of Symptoms

Some people with neuroplastic pain experience symptoms in multiple parts of their bodies. Assuming you don't have a systemic disorder such as multiple sclerosis, cystic fibrosis, or lupus, this points to neuroplastic pain. Having three or four unrelated physical conditions is extremely unlikely. A single underlying cause—neuroplastic pain—is a far more plausible explanation.

Symptoms Spread or Move

I've had patients whose pain starts in the lower-right side of their back and over time spreads to the left side. And then to the middle. Soon their entire back is in pain. When the symptoms spread over time, it's indicative of neuroplastic pain.

Likewise, sometimes neuroplastic pain bounces around from one area to another. For example, you feel pain in your left leg one day and in your right leg the next. Or you have lumbar pain in the morning and thoracic pain in the afternoon. This is not how structurally caused pain acts.

Symptoms Triggered by Stress

Does your pain get worse when you're running late for an appointment? Or when you're arguing with your spouse? Or when you send a snarky email about Tim from accounting and then realize you accidentally hit "Reply all"?

If you have pain that comes on or gets worse during times of stress, that's indicative of neuroplastic pain.

On the flip side, when you're engaged in an activity and enjoying the experience, you may find there's a decrease in your pain. Much like my Lakers story in chapter 4, this can be valuable evidence that you have neuroplastic pain.

Triggers That Have Nothing to Do with Your Body

In chapter 4, I talk about conditioned responses—instances when pain becomes linked with a neutral trigger. Often these are physical positions or activities, but sometimes our symptoms can become linked with other triggers as well. I've had patients whose pain fluctuates depending on the weather, sounds, smells, or even time of day (for example, pain that's worse in the morning or comes on only at night). One patient's pain even came on every time she watched the TV show *The Bachelor!* These are all just conditioned responses.

If your pain is triggered by something that has nothing to do with your body, that's a clear sign that it's neuroplastic.

Symmetrical Symptoms

I've had many patients who developed pain on the same part of their body on opposite sides. Both wrists, both ankles, both thumbs. It's very unusual to develop a physical problem on both sides of your body at the same time. This suggests neuroplastic pain.

Delayed Pain

Sometimes patients with neuroplastic pain experience symptoms only after they complete an activity. One of my patients had chronic lower back pain, and hiking was a big trigger for her. Except she never had pain while she was hiking. It would always come on an hour or so after she finished. This type of delayed onset is not something you see with structurally caused pain.

Childhood Adversity

People who have experienced trauma in their childhood, such as abuse or neglect, are more likely to develop chronic pain as adults.

But it isn't just *major* trauma that can lead to neuroplastic pain. Anything that made you feel unsafe growing up can predispose you to chronic pain.

Maybe you grew up with an anxious dad who always jumped to the worst-case scenario.

Maybe you had a critical mom who made you feel like you were never good enough.

Maybe your father was an alcoholic and you never knew what kind of mood he'd be in.

Maybe your mother was depressed and you were preoccupied with making her feel better.

Maybe your older sister got all the attention and you didn't get your needs met.

Or maybe your home life was relatively trauma-free, but you were bullied in seventh grade or went to an ultracompetitive high school or were ostracized on social media.

When you have these kinds of experiences growing up, it can cause you to see the world through a lens of danger, which makes you more susceptible to neuroplastic pain.

Common Personality Traits

Certain personality traits are common in people with neuroplastic pain. As I discuss in chapters 3 and 8, many pain patients are prone to self-criticism, putting pressure on themselves, and worrying. Here are some other traits that are common in neuroplastic pain patients, with a brief example of each:

- perfectionism—Bob spends twenty minutes writing a three-sentence email because he wants the tone to be *just right.*

- conscientiousness—Emily's group project is due tomorrow. She's staying up all night fixing everyone else's work to make sure they get an A.
- people-pleasing—Jennifer asks Liam to take her to the airport. Even though it's during rush hour and he has a million things to do, he says yes because he's afraid of disappointing her.
- anxiousness—Daniel never wants to be late, so he always gets to social gatherings ten minutes early. But he doesn't want to be the first one there, so he waits in his car until he sees other people going in.

It's not surprising that all these traits are associated with neuroplastic pain. Each of them puts the brain on high alert, albeit in different ways.

Lack of Physical Diagnosis

If doctors are unable to find any clear cause for your pain, that's a pretty solid indicator that it's neuroplastic. But if you *have* been given a diagnosis, don't despair. The majority of patients that I've worked with had been given a physical diagnosis at some point (and many of them more than one). As I mention in chapter 4, doctors are trained to look for structural causes. This means that sometimes they zero in on a structural issue, even if it isn't actually causing the pain.

But if you have been lucky enough to hear the words "We can't find anything wrong" from your medical practitioner, that's as clear a sign as any that your pain is neuroplastic.

Where to Go from Here

You may see yourself in some of these sections or even all of them. That's great evidence that your pain is neuroplastic. But perhaps none of these guidelines resonates with you. You may be thinking, "I don't have pain in multiple areas, and it doesn't bounce around. It's only in one place in my body, it never moves, and it's not affected by stress."

Even if none of these guidelines applies, you could still have neuroplastic pain. Neuroplastic pain is very good at mimicking structurally caused pain. As you practice the techniques outlined in this book, keep these guidelines in mind. Often patients start seeing evidence that their pain is neuroplastic as they apply the lessons of Pain Reprocessing Therapy.

Finally, another way to determine the source of your pain is to see a doctor who specializes in diagnosing neuroplastic pain. I've put together a list of physicians with this specialty at PainReprocessingTherapy.com.

Acknowledgments

First and foremost, I'd like to thank Alon Ziv, my coauthor and friend. You helped make this book immensely better, and it was really fun to write together (with the possible exception of the Chapter 3 Incident . . .).

To Richard Abate, for finding the perfect editor for the book. And to Lucia Watson, for being that editor. Your positivity and flexibility made the process feel smooth, even when it wasn't.

To the team at the Pain Psychology Center, for your hard work, your amazing talent, and your gentle indulgence of my many sports analogies.

To Tor Wager, Yoni Ashar, and the rest of the study team—we'll always have Boulder.

To Howard Schubiner, for your wisdom, your friendship, and your incessant *Columbo* references.

To John Sarno and David Schechter for teaching me about the mind-body connection.

To Dave Clarke, for your support, your generosity, and more free medical advice than I care to admit.

To Rob Munger, the man behind the movement.

To Laurie Polisky, the best neuroscientist/filmmaker I know.

And finally to Christie Uipi—you're Watson to my Crick, Pippen to my Jordan, and Joey to my Chandler. None of this would have been the same without you.

Notes

Chapter 1: This Kid's Brain Could Change the World

1 **medical talk show produced by Dr. Phil:** *The Doctors* is an Emmy Award–winning syndicated talk show that covers a wide variety of medical and health issues. Distributed domestically and internationally by CBS Television Distribution, it's a spin-off of *Dr. Phil*, which itself is a spin-off of *The Oprah Winfrey Show*.

1 **For this particular episode:** Casey and I appeared on season 9, episode 74, of *The Doctors*, which originally aired in January 2017.

2 **scan that shows brain activity:** Functional magnetic resonance imaging (fMRI) records changes in blood flow in the brain. When a part of the brain is working hard, more blood flows to that area, so fMRIs show which parts of the brain are active. Our hope was that we would see a different pattern of activity in Casey's brain once he was out of chronic pain.

6 **More than 50 million adults suffer from chronic pain in the United States:** This number comes from the Centers for Disease Control and Prevention (CDC). The CDC analyzed data from the 2016 National Health Interview Survey and determined that slightly more than 50 million American adults suffered from chronic pain, which is 20.4 percent of the population. The CDC defines "chronic pain" as "pain on most days or every day in the past 6 months." Dahlhamer, James, Jacqueline Lucas, Carla Zelaya, Richard Nahin, Sean Mackey, Lynn DeBar, Robert Kerns, Michael Von Korff, Linda Porter, and Charles Helmick. "Prevalence of chronic pain and high-impact chronic pain among adults—United States, 2016." *Morbidity and Mortality Weekly Report* 67, no. 36 (2018): 1001.

6 **Globally, the number is estimated to be 1.2 billion:** Worldwide estimates for chronic pain vary greatly. The World Health Organization (WHO) conducted a survey of primary care patients at fifteen locations in Asia, Africa, Europe, and the Americas. They found that, on average, 22 percent of adult patients suffered from what they called "persistent pain," which they defined as pain that "was present most of the time for a period of 6 months or more during the prior year." They included significant pain only when the patient had sought medical treatment, taken medication more than once, or "reported that the pain had interfered with life or activities a lot." Gureje, Oye,

Michael Von Korff, Gregory E. Simon, and Richard Gater. "Persistent pain and well-being: A World Health Organization study in primary care." *JAMA* 280, no. 2 (1998): 147–151.

At the time of this writing, the global population is estimated to be 7.7 billion people, with approximately 5.5 billion of them being adults; 22 percent of the adult population gives us 1.2 billion chronic pain sufferers worldwide.

7 **University of Pittsburgh looked into hypnosis and pain:** The University of Pittsburgh hypnosis study used a hot probe (119 degrees Fahrenheit) to trigger pain in its volunteers. The fMRIs showed brain activity in the thalamus, anterior cingulate cortex, mid-anterior insula, and parietal and prefrontal cortices. These regions of the brain are believed to be part of a network for experiencing pain. When the subjects experienced hypnotically induced pain (no hot probe), the fMRIs showed a similar pattern of brain activity. Derbyshire, Stuart W. G., Matthew G. Whalley, V. Andrew Stenger, and David A. Oakley. "Cerebral activation during hypnotically induced and imagined pain." *Neuroimage* 23, no. 1 (2004): 392–401.

8 **Back pain is the most common form of chronic pain:** The National Center for Health Statistics found the following rates of pain in its 2017 National Health Interview Survey:

Pain in lower back: 28 percent

Migraines or severe headaches: 15.5 percent

Pain in neck: 14.9 percent

Pain in face or jaw: 4.4 percent

National Center for Health Statistics. "Migraines and pain in neck, lower back, face, or jaw among adults aged 18 and over, by selected characteristics." National Health Interview Survey, 2017. Hyattsville, Maryland, 2018. Hoy, Damian, Lyn March, Peter Brooks, Fiona Blyth, Anthony Woolf, Christopher Bain, Gail Williams, et al. "The global burden of low back pain: Estimates from the Global Burden of Disease 2010 study." *Annals of the Rheumatic Diseases* 73, no. 6 (2014): 968–974.

9 **common back surgeries are simply not effective:** This study found that patients who underwent discectomies did no better than those who didn't have surgery:

Thomas, Kenneth C., Charles G. Fisher, Michael Boyd, Paul Bishop, Peter Wing, and Marcel F. Dvorak. "Outcome evaluation of surgical and nonsurgical management of lumbar disc protrusion causing radiculopathy." *Spine* 32, no. 13 (2007): 1414–1422.

This review of four separate studies showed that lumbar fusion surgery was no more effective than nonsurgical treatment:

Mirza, Sohail K., and Richard A. Deyo. "Systematic review of randomized trials comparing lumbar fusion surgery to nonoperative care for treatment of chronic back pain." *Spine* 32, no. 7 (2007): 816–823.

This review of four popular orthopedic surgeries found that none of them were more effective than placebo "sham" surgeries in reducing pain and disability:

Louw, Adriaan, Ina Diener, César Fernández-de-las-Peñas, and Emilio J. Puentedura. "Sham surgery in orthopedics: A systematic review of the literature." *Pain Medicine* 18, no. 4 (2017): 736–750.

9 **continued back pain after surgery is so common that there's even a name for it:** Failed back surgery syndrome is a very common outcome of spinal surgery. Exactly how common varies depending on which type of surgery and whom you ask (the patient or the surgeon). One study of lumbar fusion found that 46 percent of patients experienced the same level of pain or worse after surgery. Other studies have found failure rates between 19 and 36 percent.

This review gives background on failed back surgery syndrome and discusses failure rates for different surgeries:

Chan, Chin-wern, and Philip Peng. "Failed back surgery syndrome." *Pain Medicine* 12, no. 4 (2011): 577–606.

9 **64 percent of people with no back pain have disc bulges, protrusions, herniations, or disc degeneration:** The study found that 64 percent of subjects with no back pain had at least one abnormal disc, while 38 percent had more than one! Jensen, Maureen C., Michael N. Brant-Zawadzki, Nancy Obuchowski, Michael T. Modic, Dennis Malkasian, and Jeffrey S. Ross. "Magnetic resonance imaging of the lumbar spine in people without back pain." *New England Journal of Medicine* 331, no. 2 (1994): 69–73.

9 **no relationship between any of these structural issues and the subjects' symptoms:** Kleinstück, Frank, Jiri Dvorak, and Anne F. Mannion. "Are 'structural abnormalities' on magnetic resonance imaging a contraindication to the successful conservative treatment of chronic nonspecific low back pain?" *Spine* 31, no. 19 (2006): 2250–2257.

10 **scientists at Northwestern University embarked on a new frontier: predicting pain:** Baliki, Marwan N., Bogdan Petre, Souraya Torbey, Kristina M. Herrmann, Lejian Huang, Thomas J. Schnitzer, Howard L. Fields, and A. Vania Apkarian. "Corticostriatal functional

connectivity predicts transition to chronic back pain." *Nature Neuroscience* 15, no. 8 (2012): 1117–1119.

11 **no structural basis for chronic whiplash syndrome:** This article discusses the lack of structural damage in chronic whiplash and varying rates of it in different countries: Ferrari, Robert, and Anthony S. Russell. "Epidemiology of whiplash: An international dilemma." *Annals of the Rheumatic Diseases* 58, no. 1 (1999): 1–5.

11 **Chronic whiplash simply doesn't exist in Lithuania:** In the Lithuania study, almost half the subjects had some kind of pain immediately following their accident: 10 percent had neck pain, 19 percent had a headache, and an additional 18 percent had neck pain *and* a headache. Yet after one year, the percentage of subjects reporting pain had dropped to the same level as that of Lithuanians who had never been in an accident. Obelieniene, Diana, Harald Schrader, Gunnar Bovim, Irena Misevičiene, and Trond Sand. "Pain after whiplash: A prospective controlled inception cohort study." *Journal of Neurology, Neurosurgery, and Psychiatry* 66, no. 3 (1999): 279–283.

11 **Researchers in Germany conducted a brilliant and slightly crazy experiment:** Castro, W. H. M., S. J. Meyer, M. E. R. Becke, C. G. Nentwig, M. F. Hein, B. I. Ercan, S. Thomann, U. Wessels, and A. E. Du Chesne. "No stress—no whiplash?" *International Journal of Legal Medicine* 114, no. 6 (2001): 316–322.

13 **we got an fMRI of Casey's brain both before and after treatment:** Casey and I were on *The Doctors* again several months after our first appearance for a follow-up (season 9, episode 162). In this episode, Casey talks about his recovery, and we compare the results of his fMRI from before and after his treatment.

14 **sound like spells from Harry Potter:** Structures in the brain and spells in Harry Potter sound the same because they're both based on Latin. "Anterior insula" means "the front part of the island" in Latin, so I like to imagine that if Harry Potter cast this spell, it would send me to a beach in Hawaii.

14 **they're all involved in processing pain:** Bastuji, Hélène, Maud Frot, Caroline Perchet, Koichi Hagiwara, and Luis Garcia-Larrea. "Convergence of sensory and limbic noxious input into the anterior insula and the emergence of pain from nociception." *Scientific Reports* 8, no. 1 (2018): 1–9. Harris, Haley N., and Yuan B. Peng. "Evidence and explanation for the involvement of the nucleus accumbens in pain processing." *Neural Regeneration Research* 15, no. 4 (2020): 597.

15 **even involves different parts of the brain:** Apkarian, A. Vania, Javeria A. Hashmi, and Marwan N. Baliki. "Pain and the brain:

Specificity and plasticity of the brain in clinical chronic pain." *Pain* 152, no. 3 suppl. (2011): S49.

15 **unique pattern of brain activity when people experience pain:** Woo, Choong-Wan, Liane Schmidt, Anjali Krishnan, Marieke Jepma, Mathieu Roy, Martin A. Lindquist, Lauren Y. Atlas, and Tor D. Wager. "Quantifying cerebral contributions to pain beyond nociception." *Nature Communications* 8, no. 1 (2017): 1–14.

16 **a thousand miles from Los Angeles:** At the time, Dr. Wager and his lab were at the University of Colorado Boulder. Since we completed the study, they've moved to Dartmouth, which is about three thousand miles from L.A. So I guess it could have been worse.

17 **Fifty patients were randomly placed in our treatment group:** While fifty patients were randomly selected to be in the treatment group, five of them dropped out of the study before receiving a medical evaluation from Dr. Schubiner. So in the end, Christie and I treated forty-five patients with Pain Reprocessing Therapy.

18 **66 percent were Pain-Free/Nearly Pain-Free:** Ashar, Yoni K., Alan Gordon, Howard Schubiner, Christie Uipi, Karen Knight, Zachary Anderson, Judith Carlisle, Laurie Polisky, Stephan Geuter, Thomas F. Flood, Phillip A. Kragel, Sona Dimidjian, Mark A. Lumley, and Tor D. Wager. "Pain Reprocessing Therapy for Chronic Back Pain: A Randomized Controlled Trial with Functional Neuroimaging." Manuscript submitted for publication (2021).

19 **anterior insula plays an important role in deciding if the brain should generate pain:** Wiech, Katja, Chia-shu Lin, Kay H. Brodersen, Ulrike Bingel, Markus Ploner, and Irene Tracey. "Anterior insula integrates information about salience into perceptual decisions about pain." *Journal of Neuroscience* 30, no. 48 (2010): 16324–16331.

Chapter 2: Pain Is a Danger Signal

22 **fire alarm was designed to warn people of danger:** According to the *National Fire Alarm and Signaling Code* (from the National Fire Protection Association), alarms in sleeping areas should be at least seventy-five decibels "to ensure that audible public mode signals are clearly heard." Mission accomplished. This alarm was definitely clearly heard, and it was much louder than seventy-five decibels, which is about as loud as a vacuum cleaner.

Much like the fire alarm in my dorm, your brain makes sure that its danger signals are clearly heard.

23 **though pain feels simple, it's actually quite complex:** For a thorough explanation of the modern understanding of pain, I recommend this article: Moseley, G. Lorimer. "Reconceptualising pain according to modern pain science." *Physical Therapy Reviews* 12, no. 3 (2007): 169–178.

As the author says, "Pain is never really straightforward, even when it appears to be." The article is a bit technical, but the most important takeaway for our purposes is that pain is generated by the brain in an attempt to protect the body.

24 **Khrushchev's sentence was misinterpreted:** This fascinating article discusses "We will bury you!" and a few other mistranslations that may have changed history: Polizzotti, Mark. "Why mistranslation matters." *New York Times*, July 29, 2018, SR10.

25 **it processed them as pain, pain, pain:** When the construction worker arrived at the hospital, he was in so much agony that he needed to be sedated before they could take off his boot. His pain was absolutely real, but it wasn't caused by his foot; it was caused by his brain. Fisher J. P., D. T. Hassan, N. O'Connor, "Minerva." *British Medical Journal* 310 (January 7, 1995): 70.

25 **They felt pain:** Fifty percent of the subjects hooked up to the fake shock generator experienced head pain. As a further twist, the scientists put a large knob on the front of the machine. The higher the knob was turned up, the more pain the subjects reported. Even though the knob, like the shock generator, didn't actually do anything. Bayer, Timothy L., Paul E. Baer, and Charles Early. "Situational and psychophysiological factors in psychologically induced pain." *Pain* 44, no. 1 (1991): 45–50.

26 **don't need protecting for long:** Animals that are born relatively mature are known as "precocial." ("Precocial" is related to the word "precocious," which we use to describe kids who are advanced for their age.) A few animals, like the blue wildebeest, are so mature at birth that they are categorized as "superprecocial."

Some biologists theorize that this is why blue wildebeest are so common. Even though hartebeest are very similar animals, they are less precocial. A young hartebeest can't keep up with the adults in its herd until it's more than a week old. This may explain why there are one hundred times more wildebeest in the Serengeti than there are hartebeest. Hopcraft, J. Grant C., R. M. Holdo, E. Mwangomo, S. A. R. Mduma, S. J. Thirgood, M. Borner, J. M. Fryxell, H. Olff, and A. R. E. Sinclair. "Why are wildebeest the most abundant herbivore in the Serengeti ecosystem." In: Sinclair, R. E., et al. (eds.) *Serengeti IV:*

Sustaining biodiversity in a coupled human-natural system. Chicago: University of Chicago Press, 2015, p. 125.

26 **hyenas can run 30 to 35 miles per hour:** The spotted hyena has been observed chasing prey at up to 60 kilometers per hour, which is about 37 miles per hour. Mills, Gus, and Heribert Hofer. *Hyaenas: Status survey and conservation action plan.* No. 333.959 H992. IUCN, Gland (Suiza). SSC Hyaena Specialist Group, 1998.

26 **By way of comparison, Usain Bolt:** In 2009, Usain Bolt broke the world record for the 100-meter dash when he ran it in 9.58 seconds at the Berlin World Championships. (He also held the previous world record of 9.69 seconds.) The International Association of Athletics Federations measured his top speed during the race as 27.44 miles per hour. "Farewell to a legend: Usain Bolt's incredible career in numbers." *The Times* (London), August 1, 2017.

27 **big, beautiful brains:** The opposite of precocial is altricial—animals that are underdeveloped at birth and often require a lot of assistance from their parents. Humans are very altricial, but we really do have big, beautiful brains. Our brains aren't the largest in the animal kingdom (elephant and whale brains are bigger), but ours are five to seven times larger than expected for our body size. Furthermore, when it comes to things like overall number of neurons, size of the cortex (the part of the brain that does the thinking), and number of neurons in the cortex, humans are consistently at or near the top of the list. Herculano-Houzel, Suzana. "The human brain in numbers: A linearly scaled-up primate brain." *Frontiers in Human Neuroscience* 3 (2009): 31.

But let's not get too cocky. The long-finned pilot whale (which, confusingly, is a species of dolphin) has a bigger brain and more neurons than we do! Mortensen, Heidi S., Bente Pakkenberg, Maria Dam, Rune Dietz, Christian Sonne, Bjarni Mikkelsen, and Nina Eriksen. "Quantitative relationships in delphinid neocortex." *Frontiers in Neuroanatomy* 8 (2014): 132.

27 **"Neurons that fire together, wire together":** As neurons work together, they get better at working together. This is a fundamental tenet of modern neuroscience. It's known as Hebbian theory because it was first proposed by Donald Hebb, the "father of neuropsychology." Hebb, Donald O. *The Organization of Behavior.* Hoboken, NJ: Wiley and Sons, 1949.

Decades later, Carla Shatz coined the excellent summary "Neurons that fire together, wire together." Shatz, Carla J. "The developing brain." *Scientific American* 267, no. 3 (1992): 60–67.

28 **Neuroplastic pain is when the brain changes:** "Neuroplasticity" refers to the brain's ability to learn and change. It's something that humans are uniquely good at. But when the brain learns and changes in response to pain, it can become chronic. That's neuroplastic pain. Melzack, Ronald, Terence J. Coderre, Joel Katz, and Anthony L. Vaccarino. "Central neuroplasticity and pathological pain." *Annals of the New York Academy of Sciences* 933, no. 1 (2001): 157–174.

28 **shifted to parts of the brain associated with learning and memory:** Hashmi, Javeria A., Marwan N. Baliki, Lejian Huang, Alex T. Baria, Souraya Torbey, Kristina M. Hermann, Thomas J. Schnitzer, and A. Vania Apkarian. "Shape shifting pain: Chronification of back pain shifts brain representation from nociceptive to emotional circuits." *Brain* 136, no. 9 (2013): 2751–2768.

30 **Most chronic pain is neuroplastic pain:** This article is long and technical but has some good information about neuroplastic pain in various parts of the body. (Note: instead of "neuroplastic pain," the author uses the term "central sensitization," but it's the same phenomenon. "Central sensitization" refers to the idea that the central nervous system has learned to be too sensitive to pain.) Woolf, Clifford J. "Central sensitization: Implications for the diagnosis and treatment of pain." *Pain* 152, no. 3 (2011): S2–S15.

I know that even after everything you just read, it can be challenging to accept that you have neuroplastic pain. It's hard to let go of the idea that your pain is caused by a physical problem in your body. Chapter 4 can help you embrace this new perspective (which is why chapter 4 is called "Embracing a New Perspective").

Chapter 3: Nothing to Fear but Fear Itself

34 **Gandhi said that fear was our enemy:** "The enemy is fear. We think it is hate; but it is really fear." —Mahatma Gandhi: Richardson, Holly. "The blessings of Ramadan." *Salt Lake Tribune*, May 9, 2018.

34 **Mandela felt that it was a challenge to overcome:** "I learned that courage was not the absence of fear, but the triumph over it. The brave man is not he who does not feel afraid, but he who conquers that fear." —Nelson Mandela: "Mandela in his own words." CNN, June 26, 2008.

34 **"the path to the dark side":** "Fear is the path to the dark side. Fear leads to anger. Anger leads to hate. Hate leads to suffering."—Yoda: *Star Wars: Episode I—The Phantom Menace.* Directed by George Lucas. United States: Lucasfilm, 1999.

35　**Noises seem louder when we're afraid:** Siegel, Erika H., and Jeanine K. Stefanucci. "A little bit louder now: Negative affect increases perceived loudness." *Emotion* 11, no. 4 (2011): 1006.

35　**more sensitive to smell when they're on high alert:** Krusemark, Elizabeth A., and Wen Li. "Enhanced olfactory sensory perception of threat in anxiety: An event-related fMRI study." *Chemosensory Perception* 5, no. 1 (2012): 37–45.

35　**terrifying pictures and a hot probe:** Kirwilliam, S. S., and S. W. G. Derbyshire. "Increased bias to report heat or pain following emotional priming of pain-related fear." *Pain* 137, no. 1 (2008): 60–65.

35　**sometimes the participants felt pain when there was no hot pulse:** In Experiment 1 of the study, there were fifteen times when subjects reported "false pain" (pain when there was no hot pulse) when they had been looking at the scary pictures. When they had been looking at the neutral photos, they reported "false pain" zero times.

36　**stressful situations when their pain first appeared:** I'll talk more about how the modern world can put us on "high alert" (and what to do about it) in chapter 7.

36　**people who have experienced early-life stress are more sensitive to fear:** Williams, Leanne M., Justine M. Gatt, Peter R. Schofield, Gloria Olivieri, Anthony Peduto, and Evian Gordon. "'Negativity bias' in risk for depression and anxiety: Brain–body fear circuitry correlates, 5-HTT-LPR and early life stress." *Neuroimage* 47, no. 3 (2009): 804–814.

37　**worrying, putting pressure on yourself, and self-criticism:** In chapter 8, I'll discuss these three habits in more detail and outline how to gradually unlearn them.

37　**"Supposing it didn't," said Pooh:** Piglet and Pooh have this conversation during a roaring storm. After this exchange, the scene continues: "Piglet was comforted by this, and in a little while they were knocking and ringing very cheerfully at Owl's door."

We all face storms in life, and it's easy to fall into fear. I tell my patients (and myself) to remember Pooh's calm wisdom. Milne, A. A. *The House at Pooh Corner.* London: Methuen, 1928.

37　**worries . . . can increase feelings of danger and put your brain on high alert:** Engert, Veronika, Jonathan Smallwood, and Tania Singer. "Mind your thoughts: Associations between self-generated thoughts and stress-induced and baseline levels of cortisol and alpha-amylase." *Biological Psychology* 103 (2014): 283–291.

37 **Pressure puts us on high alert:** Wang, Jiongjiong, Marc Korczykowski, Hengyi Rao, Yong Fan, John Pluta, Ruben C. Gur, Bruce S. McEwen, and John A. Detre. "Gender difference in neural response to psychological stress." *Social Cognitive and Affective Neuroscience* 2, no. 3 (2007): 227–239.

38 **Claude Monet is one of the most famous painters of all time:** Claude Monet's water lilies are as iconic as Vincent van Gogh's sunflowers and Salvador Dalí's clocks. Monet was one of several artists who invented the Impressionist style, but he is often called the "father of Impressionism." After all, the movement was named after one of his paintings: *Impression, Sunrise.* Richman-Abdou, Kelly. "How this one painting sparked the Impressionist movement." My Modern Met, July 7, 2019. Retrieved from https://mymodernmet.com/claude-monet -impression-sunrise/.

38 **"I'm not a great painter":** Monet's self-critical quotes come from Kendall, Richard. *Monet by Himself: Paintings, Drawings, Pastels, Letters.* New York: Time Warner, 2004. McNearney, Allison. "When Claude Monet slashed and destroyed his own paintings." *Daily Beast,* October 29, 2017. Retrieved from https://www.thedailybeast.com/when-claude -monet-slashed-and-destroyed-his-own-paintings.

38 **French prime minister called Monet "the king of the grumps":** King, Ross. *Mad Enchantment: Claude Monet and the Painting of the Water Lilies.* New York: Bloomsbury, 2016.

38 **self-criticism . . . puts your brain on high alert:** Gruen, Rand J., Raul Silva, Joshua Ehrlich, Jack W. Schweitzer, and Arnold J. Friedhoff. "Vulnerability to stress: Self-criticism and stress-induced changes in biochemistry." *Journal of Personality* 65, no. 1 (1997): 33–47.

41 **Fear is the fuel for the pain:** Pain-related fear and its relationship with chronic pain have been studied extensively. Pain-related fear goes by different names: fear of pain, pain anxiety, pain catastrophizing (thinking extremely negative thoughts about the pain), kinesiophobia (fear of movement associated with the pain), and fear-avoidance beliefs (fear around activity and work). There is very strong evidence that pain-related fear increases pain intensity and makes pain more likely to become chronic.

41 **A study in the Netherlands showed this phenomenon:** Picavet, H. Susan J., Johan W. S. Vlaeyen, and Jan S. A. G. Schouten. "Pain catastrophizing and kinesiophobia: Predictors of chronic low back pain." *American Journal of Epidemiology* 156, no. 11 (2002): 1028–1034.

42 **dozens of studies on everything from headaches to knee pain to fibromyalgia all show the same pattern:** Headaches: Saadah, H. A. "Headache fear." *Journal of the Oklahoma State Medical Association* 90, no. 5 (1997): 179–184.

Knee pain: Kendell, Katherine, Brian Saxby, Malcolm Farrow, and Carolyn Naisby. "Psychological factors associated with short-term recovery from total knee replacement." *British Journal of Health Psychology* 6, no. 1 (2001): 41–52.

Fibromyalgia: Gupta, A., A. J. Silman, D. Ray, R. Morriss, C. Dickens, G. J. MacFarlane, Y. H. Chiu, B. Nicholl, and J. McBeth. "The role of psychosocial factors in predicting the onset of chronic widespread pain: Results from a prospective population-based study." *Rheumatology* 46, no. 4 (2007): 666–671.

Back pain: Swinkels-Meewisse, Ilse E. J., Jeffrey Roelofs, Erik G. W. Schouten, André L. M. Verbeek, Rob A. B. Oostendorp, and Johan W. S. Vlaeyen. "Fear of movement/(re)injury predicting chronic disabling low back pain: A prospective inception cohort study." *Spine* 31, no. 6 (2006): 658–664.

Neck pain: Nederhand, Marc J., Maarten J. Ijzerman, Hermie J. Hermens, Dennis C. Turk, and Gerrit Zilvold. "Predictive value of fear avoidance in developing chronic neck pain disability: Consequences for clinical decision making." *Archives of Physical Medicine and Rehabilitation* 85, no. 3 (2004): 496–501.

Back and/or neck pain: Boersma, Katja, and Steven J. Linton. "Expectancy, fear and pain in the prediction of chronic pain and disability: A prospective analysis." *European Journal of Pain* 10, no. 6 (2006): 551–557.

Shoulder pain: Parr, Jeffrey J., Paul A. Borsa, Roger B. Fillingim, Mark D. Tillman, Todd M. Manini, Chris M. Gregory, and Steven Z. George. "Pain-related fear and catastrophizing predict pain intensity and disability independently using an induced muscle injury model." *Journal of Pain* 13, no. 4 (2012): 370–378.

Pelvic pain: Glowacka, Maria, Natalie Rosen, Jill Chorney, Erna Snelgrove, and Ronald B. George. "Prevalence and predictors of genito-pelvic pain in pregnancy and postpartum: The prospective impact of fear avoidance." *Journal of Sexual Medicine* 11, no. 12 (2014): 3021–3034.

Various types of chronic pain including back pain, leg pain, neck and shoulder pain, arm pain, pelvic pain, whole body pain, head and face pain, belly pain, and chest pain: Samwel, Han J. A., Floris W.

Kraaimaat, Andrea W. M. Evers, and Ben J. P. Crul. "The role of fear-avoidance and helplessness in explaining functional disability in chronic pain: A prospective study." *International Journal of Behavioral Medicine* 14, no. 4 (2007): 237–241.

43 **downward spiral that we call the pain-fear cycle:** Chris and Molly's date and the pain-fear cycle are both examples of positive feedback loops. You know how sometimes at live events, the microphone will make that horrible whine? That's a positive feedback loop.

It starts as a small sound that gets picked up by the microphone. The small sound gets amplified and played out of the speakers. Now it's a medium sound, and it gets picked up by the microphone again. And amplified again. And played out of the speakers again. But now it's a big sound. Soon it's a huge, piercing shriek.

But my favorite example of a positive feedback loop is a cattle stampede.

We think of cows as placid animals that just stand around and eat grass all day, but don't underestimate them. Like many prey animals, cows evolved to outrun predators, and they can race up to twenty-five miles per hour. Cows are easily spooked. Something as minor as lighting a match has been known to set them off. And once one cow gets scared and starts running, the panic can spread, and soon other cows are running too.

The cows run because they're scared. The higher the level of panic, the more cows start running. And the more cows that run, the higher the level of panic. It's a classic positive feedback loop, and it often ends with the whole herd running in a stampede.

46 **We need to eliminate your fear:** Reducing pain-related fear reduces pain and disability. Smeets, Rob J. E. M., Johan W. S. Vlaeyen, Arnold D. M. Kester, and J. André Knottnerus. "Reduction of pain catastrophizing mediates the outcome of both physical and cognitive-behavioral treatment in chronic low back pain." *Journal of Pain* 7, no. 4 (2006): 261–271. De Jong, Jeroen R., Karoline Vangronsveld, Madelon L. Peters, Mariëlle E. J. B. Goossens, Patrick Onghena, Isis Bulté, and Johan W. S. Vlaeyen. "Reduction of pain-related fear and disability in post-traumatic neck pain: A replicated single-case experimental study of exposure in vivo." *Journal of Pain* 9, no. 12 (2008): 1123–1134.

De Jong, Jeroen R., Johan W. S. Vlaeyen, Marjon van Eijsden, Christoph Loo, and Patrick Onghena. "Reduction of pain-related fear and increased function and participation in work-related upper extremity pain (WRUEP): Effects of exposure in vivo." *Pain* 153, no. 10 (2012): 2109–2118.

Chapter 4: Embracing a New Perspective

49 **movie where Brad Pitt ages backward:** *The Curious Case of Benjamin Button*. Directed by David Fincher. United States: Paramount Pictures, 2008.

50 **You might remember:** Dr. Howard Schubiner is a board-certified internal medicine specialist. He is the founder and director of the Mind Body Medicine Program at Ascension Providence Hospital and a Clinical Professor at Michigan State University.

51 **exact fear that fuels neuroplastic pain:** As I mentioned in chapter 2, pain is designed to warn us that there's a problem in the body. So the belief that pain has a physical cause is natural, and we all have it. But when this belief is especially strong, it leads to excess fear, which fuels neuroplastic pain.

This has been studied extensively by scientists. They measure how strong this belief is with questionnaires that ask fun stuff like "How strongly do you agree with this statement? 'Pain is my body telling me I have something dangerously wrong.'" Studies on everything from back pain to neck pain to knee pain all show the same thing: people who score high are more likely to develop chronic pain. Swinkels-Meewisse, Ilse E. J., Jeffrey Roelofs, Erik G. W. Schouten, André L. M. Verbeek, Rob A. B. Oostendorp, and Johan W. S. Vlaeyen. "Fear of movement/(re)injury predicting chronic disabling low back pain: A prospective inception cohort study." *Spine* 31, no. 6 (2006): 658–664. Nederhand, Marc J., Maarten J. Ijzerman, Hermie J. Hermens, Dennis C. Turk, and Gerrit Zilvold. "Predictive value of fear avoidance in developing chronic neck pain disability: Consequences for clinical decision making." *Archives of Physical Medicine and Rehabilitation* 85, no. 3 (2004): 496–501. Helminen, Eeva-Eerika, Sanna H. Sinikallio, Anna L. Valjakka, Rauni H. Väisänen-Rouvali, and Jari P. A. Arokoski. "Determinants of pain and functioning in knee osteoarthritis: A one-year prospective study." *Clinical Rehabilitation* 30, no. 9 (2016): 890–900.

A study in Holland measured people's belief that pain reflects damage in the body. Then they followed up with the subjects six months later. The scientists found some interesting trends in the participants who scored high for this type of belief.

Some high-belief subjects started the study with back pain. They were much more likely to still have back pain at the follow-up than were people who scored lower on structural belief. Believing that their pain was caused by a structural problem kept their pain stuck.

Other high-belief subjects had no back pain at the beginning of the study. But they were also much more likely to have back pain at the follow-up than their low-belief peers were. A strong belief that pain is always a sign of physical damage made new pain more likely. Picavet, H. Susan J., Johan W. S. Vlaeyen, and Jan S. A. G. Schouten. "Pain catastrophizing and kinesiophobia: Predictors of chronic low back pain." *American Journal of Epidemiology* 156, no. 11 (2002): 1028–1034.

51 **And soon after, the pain fades:** The good news is that when patients are able to reduce their belief that their pain is caused by physical damage, their pain improves. Doménech, Julio, Vicente Sanchis-Alfonso, and Begona Espejo. "Changes in catastrophizing and kinesiophobia are predictive of changes in disability and pain after treatment in patients with anterior knee pain." *Knee Surgery, Sports Traumatology, Arthroscopy* 22, no. 10 (2014): 2295–2300. Cai, Libai, Huanhuan Gao, Huiping Xu, Yanyan Wang, Peihua Lyu, and Yanjin Liu. "Does a program based on cognitive behavioral therapy affect kinesiophobia in patients following total knee arthroplasty? A randomized, controlled trial with a 6-month follow-up." *Journal of Arthroplasty* 33, no. 3 (2018): 704–710. Guck, Thomas P., Raymond V. Burke, Christopher Rainville, Dreylana Hill-Taylor, and Dustin P. Wallace. "A brief primary care intervention to reduce fear of movement in chronic low back pain patients." *Translational Behavioral Medicine* 5, no. 1 (2015): 113–121.

52 **Pete refused to let his body heal:** Pete Reiser was considered by many of his contemporaries to be the best baseball player they'd ever seen. His first major league manager, Leo Durocher, said that Reiser was "every bit as good" as the great Willie Mays: "Pete had more power than Willie—left-handed and right-handed both . . . He had everything but luck."

But it wasn't luck that cut Reiser's career short; it was his propensity for injury and then ignoring those injuries. During his time as a player, he ran into the outfield wall eleven times! But he just kept playing, despite skull fractures and concussions. In fact, Reiser's repeatedly running into concrete walls and bare fences is the reason baseball stadiums installed padded outfield walls. Durocher, Leo. *Nice Guys Finish Last*. New York: Pocket Books, 1976. "Reckless Reiser dead at 62." *Windsor Star,* October 27, 1981.

53 **had a crippling panic attack:** Martin, Steve. *Born Standing Up: A Comic's Life*. New York: Simon & Schuster, 2008.

54 **pain isn't caused by the position or activity:** This experiment shows that pain can be a conditioned response to a neutral stimulus: Madden,

Victoria J., Valeria Bellan, Leslie N. Russek, Danny Camfferman, Johan W. S. Vlaeyen, and G. Lorimer Moseley. "Pain by association? Experimental modulation of human pain thresholds using classical conditioning." *Journal of Pain* 17, no. 10 (2016): 1105–1115.

55 **it isn't the sitting, or standing, or walking that's causing your pain:** This review looks at seven separate studies to explore the relationship between chronic pain and conditioned responses: Harvie, Daniel S., G. Lorimer Moseley, Susan L. Hillier, and Ann Meulders. "Classical conditioning differences associated with chronic pain: A systematic review." *Journal of Pain* 18, no. 8 (2017): 889–898.

56 **Doctors are trained to look for structural causes:** In medical school, future doctors learn how to diagnose diseases based on the patient's symptoms. A popular mnemonic device to help med students remember the possible causes of a disease is VINDICATE:

V—vascular

I—infection

N—neoplasm (a fancy word for a tumor)

D—degenerative

I—intoxication

C—congenital

A—autoimmune

T—trauma

E—endocrine (hormones)

This mnemonic is clearly rooted in the biomedical model. Every item on the list is physical. Doctors are trained to look for structural causes. And when you look for structural issues, you'll find some, even if they aren't actually causing the problem.

56 **Many chronic pain sufferers have been given diagnoses:** Of chronic pain sufferers, 90 percent have consulted some type of medical professional to try to ease their pain, and 38 percent have seen more than one. Most of those practitioners will take a biomedical approach that won't work. It won't help with the pain, but it will reinforce their patients' belief that they have a physical problem (which ironically will make their pain worse). Peter D. Hart Research Associates. *Americans talk about pain*, 2003, https://www .researchamerica.org/sites/default/files/uploads/poll2003pain.pdf.

56 **downside to these medical diagnoses:** The good news is that the medical community is (slowly) adopting a more holistic approach,

known as the biopsychosocial model. This approach includes the biological factors of the biomedical model but also takes psychological and social elements into account. Engel, George L. "The need for a new medical model: A challenge for biomedicine." *Science* 196, no. 4286 (1977): 129–136.

Chapter 5: Somatic Tracking

65 **The first time I watched *The Wizard of Oz*:** *The Wizard of Oz* is a cultural touchstone. According to the Library of Congress, it's the most watched movie of all time. And it coined the phrase "There's no place like home." *The Wizard of Oz*. Directed by Victor Fleming. United States: Metro-Goldwyn-Mayer, 1939.

Surprisingly, some scholars think that the movie is a political allegory about American politics of the 1890s. Supposedly, the yellow brick road represents money being backed by the gold standard. (How do we measure gold? In ounces, which we abbreviate as "oz.") "*The Wizard of Oz*: An American fairy tale." Retrieved from https://www.loc.gov /exhibits/oz/ozsect2.html. Littlefield, Henry M. "*The Wizard of Oz*: Parable on populism." *American Quarterly* 16, no. 1 (1964): 47–58.

66 **the way we do that is called somatic tracking:** "Somatic" means having to do with the body. Somatic tracking is a way to track physical sensations in your body through a new lens. This allows you to gradually change the way your brain interprets these sensations.

67 **"paying attention, on purpose, in the present moment, non-judgmentally":** Szalavitz, Maia. "Q&A: Jon Kabat-Zinn talks about bringing mindfulness meditation to medicine." *Time,* January 11, 2012.

67 **by deactivating the brain's fear circuits:** Mindfulness has been shown to reduce activity in the amygdala, an almond-shaped structure in the brain that plays a key role in experiencing fear. Doll, Anselm, Britta K. Hölzel, Satja Mulej Bratec, Christine C. Boucard, Xiyao Xie, Afra M. Wohlschläger, and Christian Sorg. "Mindful attention to breath regulates emotions via increased amygdala–prefrontal cortex connectivity." *Neuroimage* 134 (2016): 305–313.

67 **This disrupts the pain-fear cycle:** Mindfulness can help reduce neuroplastic pain. Khoo, Eve-Ling, Rebecca Small, Wei Cheng, Taylor Hatchard, Brittany Glynn, Danielle B. Rice, Becky Skidmore, Samantha Kenny, Brian Hutton, and Patricia A. Poulin. "Comparative evaluation of group-based mindfulness-based stress reduction and cognitive behavioural therapy for the treatment and management of chronic pain: A systematic review and network meta-analysis." *Evidence-Based Mental Health* 22, no. 1 (2019): 26–35.

67 safety reappraisal, has been shown by scientists to significantly decrease fear: Sloan, Tracy, and Michael J. Telch. "The effects of safety-seeking behavior and guided threat reappraisal on fear reduction during exposure: An experimental investigation." *Behaviour Research and Therapy* 40, no. 3 (2002): 235–251. Shore, Tim, Kathrin Cohen Kadosh, Miriam Lommen, Myra Cooper, and Jennifer Y. F. Lau. "Investigating the effectiveness of brief cognitive reappraisal training to reduce fear in adolescents." *Cognition and Emotion* 31, no. 4 (2017): 806–815.

68 Scientists study positive affect: Uhrig, Meike K., Nadine Trautmann, Ulf Baumgärtner, Rolf-Detlef Treede, Florian Henrich, Wolfgang Hiller, and Susanne Marschall. "Emotion elicitation: A comparison of pictures and films." *Frontiers in Psychology* 7 (2016): 180. Westermann, Rainer, Kordelia Spies, Günter Stahl, and Friedrich W. Hesse. "Relative effectiveness and validity of mood induction procedures: A meta-analysis." *European Journal of Social Psychology* 26, no. 4 (1996): 557–580.

68 when people's moods are lightened, they are better at overcoming pain-related fear: Geschwind, Nicole, Michel Meulders, Madelon L. Peters, Johan W. S. Vlaeyen, and Ann Meulders. "Can experimentally induced positive affect attenuate generalization of fear of movement-related pain?" *Journal of Pain* 16, no. 3 (2015): 258–269. Goli, Zahra, Ali Asghari, and Alireza Moradi. "Effects of mood induction on the pain responses in patients with migraine and the role of pain catastrophizing." *Clinical Psychology and Psychotherapy* 23, no. 1 (2016): 66–76.

71 Here's a quick dose of lightness to help you: We showed this photo to my coauthor's six-year-old daughter and asked her how it made her feel. She said, "Like the sun is shining inside of me." That's exactly the mood we're going for!

72 They watched it like a hawk: The idioms "watch like a hawk" and "eagle-eyed" are based in reality. Birds of prey, like hawks, eagles, and kites, are estimated to have vision that's four to eight times as powerful as humans'. They can see farther than we can, can detect movement better than we can, and are even better at distinguishing colors in some situations.

Of course, when I talk about hawk mode, I'm not referring to how well a hawk sees, but to the intensity of its gaze. Hawks have such a piercing stare because they have a large, feathered superciliary ridge (the bone above the eye sockets—we have it too). This supersize brow ridge helps shade their eyes from the sun and protect them from dust and wind. It also makes hawks look super tough, but I'm not sure if that's an official reason or just a bonus.

Bottom line: hawks can't help being intense—they're built that way. But you can. Do your best to lower your intensity when you practice somatic tracking.

Jones, Michael P., Kenneth E. Pierce Jr., and Daniel Ward. "Avian vision: A review of form and function with special consideration to birds of prey." *Journal of Exotic Pet Medicine* 16, no. 2 (2007): 69–87. Potier, Simon, Mindaugas Mitkus, and Almut Kelber. "High resolution of colour vision, but low contrast sensitivity in a diurnal raptor." *Proceedings of the Royal Society B: Biological Sciences* 285, no. 1885 (2018): 1036. Kirschbaum, Kari. "Family Accipitridae." *AnimalDiversity Web*. University of Michigan Museum of Zoology.

76 **he ended up winning two national championships in a row:** My father, Stan Gordon Tarshis (lucky for me, he dropped the Tarshis before I was born), won the NCAA championship in high bar in 1959 and 1960. If he had also won in 1958, he would have been the first three-time winner in this category. Sadly, he only got the silver that year because he lost to—you guessed it—Abie Grossfeld. "Southern California Jewish Sports Hall of Fame." 2016. Retrieved from http://scjewishsportshof.com/tarshis.html.

78 **one song I've always loved:** "The Gambler" was written by Don Schlitz in 1976. It was recorded by Schlitz and several other country music singers, but it was Kenny Rogers's version that hit number 1 on the *Billboard* Country Music charts and even crossed over to make it to number 16 on the Pop chart and number 3 on the Easy Listening chart. Whitburn, Joel. *The Billboard Book of Top 40 Country Hits: 1944–2006*. Record Research, 2004.

Chapter 6: The Process

79 **called Hinkie "a fraud," "a dunce," and "a moron":** Burneko, Albert. "The 76ers are run by a ridiculous TED-humping moron." *Deadspin*, February 18, 2015. Retrieved from https://deadspin.com/the-76ers -are-run-by-a-ridiculous-ted-humping-moron-1686613279.

80 **"Trust the process":** For a detailed history of how "Trust the process" became the unofficial catchphrase of the Philadelphia 76ers, see Rappaport, Max. "The definitive history of 'trust the process.'" *Bleacher Report*, August 23, 2017. Retrieved from https://bleacherreport .com/articles/2729018-the-definitive-history-of-trust-the-process.

80 **more wins than they'd had in seventeen years:** Unsurprisingly, the NBA does not like the idea of teams intentionally losing for multiple years. Largely in response to Hinkie's process, the NBA changed the rules of the annual draft so that there is less of an advantage for

last-place teams. Thottakara, Arun. "Tearing up the process: The NBA's new draft lottery reform seeks to counter tanking." *Villanova Sports Law Society Blog*, 2018. Retrieved from https://www1.villanova .edu/villanova/law/academics/sportslaw/commentary/sls_blog/2018 /tearing-up-the-process—the-nbas-new-draft-lottery-reform-seeks -.html.

81 **exposure to the thing you're afraid of:** Marks, Isaac. "Exposure therapy for phobias and obsessive-compulsive disorders." *Hospital Practice* 14, no. 2 (1979): 101–108. Myers, Karyn M., and Michael Davis. "Mechanisms of fear extinction." *Molecular Psychiatry* 12, no. 2 (2007): 120–150.

82 **it's a corrective experience:** Foa, Edna B., and Michael J. Kozak. "Emotional processing of fear: Exposure to corrective information." *Psychological Bulletin* 99, no. 1 (1986): 20.

84 **when exposure triggers feelings of danger:** A recent study in Texas accidentally showed setbacks in action. The researchers recruited people with agoraphobia, an anxiety disorder that can be triggered by feeling trapped in public spaces. The scientists were hoping to help the participants overcome their fear through exposure. They had the participants spend time in spaces that triggered their fear—public transportation, movie theaters, shopping malls. The goal was for the participants to have corrective experiences and reduce their fear.

But some of the participants experienced more fear during their exposure. Instead of corrective experiences, they had setbacks. And those participants had the most fear at the end of the study. Meuret, Alicia E., Anke Seidel, Benjamin Rosenfield, Stefan G. Hofmann, and David Rosenfield. "Does fear reactivity during exposure predict panic symptom reduction?" *Journal of Consulting and Clinical Psychology* 80, no. 5 (2012): 773.

86 **avoidance behaviors are an effective tool for overcoming fear:** As I mentioned earlier in the chapter, the only way to overcome a fear is through exposure. For this reason, avoidance behaviors sometimes get a bad rap. But recently, psychologists have started to realize the value of avoidance behaviors as a tool to help overcome fear. Hofmann, Stefan G., and Aleena C. Hay. "Rethinking avoidance: Toward a balanced approach to avoidance in treating anxiety disorders." *Journal of Anxiety Disorders* 55 (2018): 14–21. LeDoux, Joseph E., Justin Moscarello, Robert Sears, and Vincent Campese. "The birth, death and resurrection of avoidance: A reconceptualization of a troubled paradigm." *Molecular Psychiatry* 22, no. 1 (2017): 24–36.

Avoidance behaviors are a critical part of the Process because they can help you minimize setbacks.

86 **Avoidance behaviors are really common with chronic pain patients:** Volders, Stéphanie, Yannick Boddez, Steven De Peuter, Ann Meulders, and Johan W. S. Vlaeyen. "Avoidance behavior in chronic pain research: A cold case revisited." *Behaviour Research and Therapy* 64 (2015): 31–37.

87 **think about your own avoidance behaviors:** Because avoidance behaviors are often physical, they can reinforce the belief that your pain is caused by a problem in your body, even when it isn't. For example, if you have pain when sitting, standing up can be an effective avoidance behavior. This might cause you to think, "Oh, standing up took some strain off my spine." But if you have neuroplastic pain, your spine is irrelevant. As I discussed in chapter 4, you feel pain when you sit because it's a conditioned response. And you feel better when you stand because you're avoiding the conditioned response. Standing is not taking strain off your spine; it's making your brain feel safe.

88 **Their favorite is Chutes and Ladders:** Chutes and Ladders was first published in the United States in 1943 by Milton Bradley. Slesin, Suzanne. "At 50, still climbing, still sliding." *New York Times*, July 15, 1993, C3.

88 **A setback is like a chute:** It's worth noting that Chutes and Ladders is based on an ancient board game from India called Snakes and Ladders. This metaphor works even better with the original version, since snakes feel innately dangerous.

91 **it's common to have thoughts of fear and hopelessness:** When people have extreme negative thoughts about pain (known as pain catastrophizing), they experience more pain. George, Steven Z., and Adam T. Hirsh. "Psychologic influence on experimental pain sensitivity and clinical pain intensity for patients with shoulder pain." *Journal of Pain* 10, no. 3 (2009): 293–299.

92 **Your brain is feeling danger, and you're calming it with messages of safety:** This study found that negative thoughts made patients more sensitive to pain, but messages of safety made them less sensitive to pain: Roditi, Daniela, Michael E. Robinson, and Nola Litwins. "Effects of coping statements on experimental pain in chronic pain patients." *Journal of Pain Research* 2 (2009): 109.

98 **Harvard psychologist named B. F. Skinner:** Fun fact: The "B" stands for "Burrhus."

98 **even teaching a couple of pigeons to play Ping-Pong:** Skinner rewarded the pigeons with a food treat every time the ball got past their opponent. With this positive reinforcement, the pigeons got pretty good at hitting the ball back and forth. It's a fun mental image,

but you should know that the pigeons didn't use paddles. They knocked the ball back and forth with their beaks. You can see them in action here: https://www.youtube.com/watch?v=vGazyH6fQQ4.

98 **experiment involved placing a rat inside an enclosed chamber:** The official name for this setup is "operant conditioning chamber," but it's more commonly referred to as a Skinner box, after the man who made it famous.

98 **there was an unexpected twist—the contraption broke:** It was an accidental discovery, but Skinner immediately realized its importance: "My first extinction curve showed up by accident. A rat was pressing the lever in an experiment on satiation when the pellet dispenser jammed. I was not there at the time, and when I returned I found a beautiful curve. The rat had gone on pressing although no pellets were received . . . I was terribly excited. It was a Friday afternoon and there was no one in the laboratory who I could tell. All that weekend I crossed streets with particular care and avoided all unnecessary risks to protect my discovery from loss through my accidental death." Skinner, Burrhus Frederic. *The Shaping of a Behaviorist: Part Two of an Autobiography.* New York: Alfred A. Knopf, 1979, p. 95.

98 **This is called extinction:** It's not every day I get to cite an eighty-year-old study: Skinner, B. F. "On the rate of extinction of a conditioned reflex." *Journal of General Psychology* 8, no. 1 (1933): 114–129.

98 **This is called an extinction burst:** As I mentioned earlier, Skinner and his contemporaries described how animals responded to extinction and plotted this behavior on graphs. For example, how often a rat pressed the lever once it no longer got food as a reward. These "extinction curves" showed a gradual tapering off as the rat unlearned the behavior. But sometimes there was an increase in the behavior before it tapered off.

Fred Keller and William Schoenfeld were the first to describe this increase in activity as a "burst" in their seminal 1950 textbook, *Principles of Psychology.* They wrote, "The extinction curve shows a burst of responses." Or a little more colorfully, "The animal is apt to attack vigorously the now-unrewarding bar."

You may experience an extinction burst, but stay the course. Much like those rats eventually gave up, your pain will give up once it's not getting reinforced anymore. Keller, F. S., and W. N. Schoenfeld. *Principles of psychology: A systematic text in the science of behavior. Century Psychology Series.* East Norwalk, CT: Appleton-Century-Crofts, 1950.

Chapter 7: Breaking the High-Alert Habit

106 **35 percent of people worldwide said they had stress:** The statistics on stress worldwide and in the United States come from the Gallup 2019 Global Emotions Report. This survey is based on 151,000 interviews on positive and negative emotions conducted in 143 countries.

When asked, "Did you experience stress during a lot of the day yesterday?" 55 percent of Americans said yes. The United States tied with Albania, Iran, and Sri Lanka. We were only four points behind the most stressed country in the world, Greece, which has been mired in a devastating economic crisis for a decade.

Ray, Julie. "Americans' stress, worry and anger intensified in 2018." April 25, 2019. Gallup Organization. Retrieved from https://news .gallup.com/poll/249098/americans-stress-worry-anger-intensified -2018.aspx. Kitsantonis, Niki. "Greece, 10 years into economic crisis, counts the cost to mental health." *New York Times,* February 3, 2019. Retrieved from https://www.nytimes.com/2019/02/03/world/europe /greece-economy-mental-health.html.

107 **His brain triggers the release of stress hormones:** Jansen, Arthur S. P., Xay Van Nguyen, Vladimir Karpitskiy, Thomas C. Mettenleiter, and Arthur D. Loewy. "Central command neurons of the sympathetic nervous system: Basis of the fight-or-flight response." *Science* 270, no. 5236 (1995): 644–646.

107 **Neil's existence on the savanna is mostly calm:** Sapolsky, Robert M. *Why Zebras Don't Get Ulcers: The Acclaimed Guide to Stress, Stress-Related Diseases, and Coping.* New York: Henry Holt, 2004.

108 **seventy-two different flavors of Oreos:** The truth is that it's hard to get an exact count on the number of Oreo types because there are so many seasonal flavors (Pumpkin Spice Oreos), limited-edition flavors (Marshmallow Moon Oreos for the fiftieth anniversary of the moon landing), and international flavors (Matcha Green Tea Oreos from Japan). That said, I'm confident there are at least seventy-two distinct flavors, not even counting all the versions that just have different amounts of cream filling (Double Stuf Oreos, Mega Stuf Oreos, and the jaw-breaking Most Stuf Oreos).

This article from a couple of years ago ranks fifty-five different Oreo flavors: Ceron, Ella. "Here's every Oreo flavor ever created." *Teen Vogue,* June 19, 2017. Retrieved from https://www.teenvogue.com /story/every-oreo-flavor-ranked.

108 **We're wired to seek out things that stimulate us:** De Oca, Beatrice M., and Alison A. Black. "Bullets versus burgers: Is it threat or

relevance that captures attention?" *American Journal of Psychology* 126, no. 3 (2013): 287–300.

110 **a way to make even stronger habits:** intermittent reinforcement: Skinner, Burrhus F. "Reinforcement today." *American Psychologist* 13, no. 3 (1958): 94.

110 **Skinner basically built a rat slot machine:** The type of reinforcement used by slot machines is called "variable ratio." This means that the probability of winning is constant, but the actual number of pulls required to win is variable. For example, a slot machine may pay out on average every one hundred spins. But that's just the average. The actual number of spins required to get a jackpot will vary. Hurlburt, Russell T., Terry J. Knapp, and Steven H. Knowles. "Simulated slot-machine play with concurrent variable ratio and random ratio schedules of reinforcement." *Psychological Reports* 47, no. 2 (1980): 635–639.

110 **When the rats or gamblers "win," their neurons release a chemical called dopamine:** Winstanley, Catharine A., Paul J. Cocker, and Robert D. Rogers. "Dopamine modulates reward expectancy during performance of a slot machine task in rats: Evidence for a 'near-miss' effect." *Neuropsychopharmacology* 36, no. 5 (2011): 913–925. Joutsa, Juho, Jarkko Johansson, Solja Niemelä, Antti Ollikainen, Mika M. Hirvonen, Petteri Piepponen, Eveliina Arponen, et al. "Mesolimbic dopamine release is linked to symptom severity in pathological gambling." *Neuroimage* 60, no. 4 (2012): 1992–1999.

110 **can also create addictions—cocaine works by boosting dopamine in the brain:** Ritz, Mary C., Richard J. Lamb, and M. J. Kuhar. "Cocaine receptors on dopamine transporters are related to self -administration of cocaine." *Science* 237, no. 4819 (1987): 1219–1223.

110 **Gamblers also have elevated levels of one of the stress hormones we talked about earlier—cortisol:** Meyer, Gerhard, Berthold P. Hauffa, Manfred Schedlowski, Cornelius Pawlak, Michael A. Stadler, and Michael S. Exton. "Casino gambling increases heart rate and salivary cortisol in regular gamblers." *Biological Psychiatry* 48, no. 9 (2000): 948-953. Meyer, Gerhard, Jan Schwertfeger, Michael S. Exton, Onno E. Janssen, Wolfram Knapp, Michael A. Stadler, Manfred Schedlowski, and Tillmann H. C. Krüger. "Neuroendocrine response to casino gambling in problem gamblers." *Psychoneuroendocrinology* 29, no. 10 (2004): 1272–1280.

111 **cell phones also make our brains release dopamine:** Stone, Madeline. "Smartphone addiction now has a clinical name." *Business Insider,* July 31, 2014. Retrieved from http://www.businessinsider.com /what-is-nomophobia-2014-7?IR=T.

111 **cortisol levels go up whenever you hear your phone or even think you hear it:** Price, Catherine. "Putting down your phone may help you live longer." *New York Times*, April 24, 2019. Retrieved from https://www.nytimes.com/2019/04/24/well/mind/putting-down-your-phone-may-help-you-live-longer.html.

111 **Eighty-nine percent of people in one study had experienced "phantom vibrations":** Drouin, Michelle, Daren H. Kaiser, and Daniel A. Miller. "Phantom vibrations among undergraduates: Prevalence and associated psychological characteristics." *Computers in Human Behavior* 28, no. 4 (2012): 1490–1496.

This phenomenon is so common that there's even a Wikipedia page devoted to "phantom vibration syndrome" with some pretty great nicknames for it, like ringxiety and phonetom. See https://en.wikipedia.org/wiki/Phantom_vibration_syndrome.

111 **average person checks their smartphone 221 times per day:** "Tecmark survey finds average user picks up their smartphone 221 times a day." Tecmark, 2014. Retrieved from https://www.tecmark.co.uk/blog/smartphone-usage-data-uk-2014.

112 **In her book,** *Bossypants:* Fey, Tina. *Bossypants.* New York: Little, Brown, 2011, p. 274.

113 **safety reappraisal that can be really effective in the face of uncertainty:** Uncertainty can be stressful. In fact, sometimes the uncertainty is worse than the thing we're worried about. Some scientists in London demonstrated this with a very clever experiment. The participants in this study played a video game in which they turned over rocks. Sometimes there was a snake hiding under the rock, and sometimes there wasn't. Just to up the stakes, if there was a snake under the rock, the participant got a mild electric shock. What a fun game!

The researchers measured the participants' stress levels the whole time they were playing. Here's the interesting twist: Sometimes the participants knew for sure that there was a snake under the rock. But sometimes they just thought there might be a hidden snake.

When the participants knew for certain that they would get a shock, their stress levels went up. That makes sense. Knowing you're about to get shocked is stressful. But when the participants weren't sure if there was a snake, their stress levels went up even higher! A bad thing that might happen was more stressful than a bad thing that was definitely happening.

But as I explained in chapter 5, safety reappraisal is an effective technique for reducing fear. I predict that the people playing the snake video game could have lowered their stress levels by telling themselves,

"I might get a small shock or I might not. But it's going to be okay either way." De Berker, Archy O., Robb B. Rutledge, Christoph Mathys, Louise Marshall, Gemma F. Cross, Raymond J. Dolan, and Sven Bestmann. "Computations of uncertainty mediate acute stress responses in humans." *Nature Communications* 7, article no. 10996 (2016).

115 **Feeling trapped interferes with the Process and injects extra danger into your brain:** As I said in chapter 6, exposure is the key to overcoming fear. But exposure in a way that makes you feel unsafe leads to setbacks. Feeling trapped is a sure way to feel unsafe and put your brain on high alert.

Neuroscientist Joseph LeDoux has done interesting work in this area and has shown that feeling trapped and out of control increases fear. But as LeDoux recently wrote, "When the person gains control of situations through their own actions, anxiety diminishes." Boeke, Emily A., Justin M. Moscarello, Joseph E. LeDoux, Elizabeth A. Phelps, and Catherine A. Hartley. "Active avoidance: Neural mechanisms and attenuation of Pavlovian conditioned responding." *Journal of Neuroscience* 37, no. 18 (2017): 4808–4818. LeDoux, Joseph. "For the anxious, avoidance can have an upside." *New York Times*, April 7, 2013. Retrieved from https://opinionator.blogs.nytimes.com/2013 /04/07/for-the-anxious-avoidance-can-have-an-upside.

Do what you can to take control of your own situations and avoid feeling trapped. This will reduce your fear and your pain.

Chapter 8: Getting Good at Feeling Good

121 **"The Tale of Two Wolves":** Like most parables, "The Tale of Two Wolves" has dozens of different versions, and it's difficult to figure out its exact origin. It's often presented as a Cherokee legend, but there's no evidence that it has any Native American connection. Some believe that the first example of its use was in a book by the Christian evangelist Billy Graham. His version doesn't have wolves or a wise grandfather. It's about two fighting dogs (one black, one white) owned by an "Eskimo fisherman." But it has the same moral: "The one I feed always wins because he is stronger." Graham, Billy. *The Holy Spirit: Activating God's Power in Your Life.* Nashville: W Publishing Group, 1978, p. 92.

122 **Positive emotions soothe your pain:** This review explores the relationship between "positive affect" and pain. Positive emotions can reduce both experimentally induced pain (electric shocks, hot probes) and chronic pain: Finan, Patrick H., and Eric L. Garland. "The role of positive affect in pain and its treatment." *Clinical Journal of Pain* 31, no. 2 (2015): 177.

126 **This technique is called "catching your fears" and it's a simple three-step process:** Catching your fears is a version of "cognitive restructuring"—a technique designed to reduce negative thoughts and replace them with positive ones. A large body of evidence shows that cognitive restructuring is effective at reducing various types of fear, including pain-related fear. Mattick, Richard P., Lorna Peters, and J. Christopher Clarke. "Exposure and cognitive restructuring for social phobia: A controlled study." *Behavior Therapy* 20, no. 1 (1989): 3–23. De Jongh, A. D., Peter Muris, Guusje Ter Horst, Florence Van Zuuren, Nelleke Schoenmakers, and Peter Makkes. "One-session cognitive treatment of dental phobia: Preparing dental phobics for treatment by restructuring negative cognitions." *Behaviour Research and Therapy* 33, no. 8 (1995): 947–954. Watt, Margo C., Sherry H. Stewart, Marie-Josée Lefaivre, and Lindsay S. Uman. "A brief cognitive-behavioral approach to reducing anxiety sensitivity decreases pain-related anxiety." *Cognitive Behaviour Therapy* 35, no. 4 (2006): 248–256.

To study the effectiveness of catching fears, some scientists recruited people who suffer from test anxiety. Now, nobody likes taking tests, but for people with test anxiety, "All of the above" is the stuff of nightmares. As part of the study, the participants had to take some tests, but first they practiced catching any fears that came up. And it worked! By catching their fears, they became less scared of tests. But the really cool part is that by the end of the study, the subjects also had less fear of other situations, like giving a speech, going to a party, and interviewing for a job. By catching their negative thoughts around tests, they lowered their fear across the board. Goldfried, Marvin R., Marsha M. Linehan, and Jean L. Smith. "Reduction of test anxiety through cognitive restructuring." *Journal of Consulting and Clinical Psychology* 46, no. 1 (1978): 32.

126 **when pain patients catch their fears, their pain decreases:** Ehde, Dawn M., and Mark P. Jensen. "Feasibility of a cognitive restructuring intervention for treatment of chronic pain in persons with disabilities." *Rehabilitation Psychology* 49, no. 3 (2004): 254. Kohl, Annika, Winfried Rief, and Julia Anna Glombiewski. "Do fibromyalgia patients benefit from cognitive restructuring and acceptance? An experimental study." *Journal of Behavior Therapy and Experimental Psychiatry* 45, no. 4 (2014): 467–474.

130 **Sometimes the doing comes first and the believing comes later:** The relationship between thoughts and beliefs is a chicken-and-egg situation. Beliefs certainly influence what we think, but what we think can also mold our beliefs. In one study, young athletes were trained in various tennis skills. Half the participants were also taught to send themselves positive messages. The positive-messages group's beliefs

about their ability to perform increased as a result of their self-talk. Their tennis performance also improved. The control group, which didn't use positive messages, had no change in their beliefs or their tennis. Hatzigeorgiadis, Antonis, Nikos Zourbanos, Christos Goltsios, and Yannis Theodorakis. "Investigating the functions of self-talk: The effects of motivational self-talk on self-efficacy and performance in young tennis players." *Sport Psychologist* 22, no. 4 (2008): 458–471.

131 **If you have chronic pain, your brain is good at experiencing negative feelings:** In the Boulder Back Pain Study, they tested this phenomenon by playing an unpleasant sound while participants were in the fMRI machine. I heard the sound, and it's pretty bad. It's a knife scraping a glass bottle, and it definitely has that fingernails-on-a-chalkboard quality. No one liked it, but chronic pain patients had a stronger response to the sound than patients in a pain-free control group. The pain patients showed increased brain activity and rated the sound as being more unpleasant. Yoni Ashar, email message to author, February 5, 2020.

132 **Even this guy:** My coauthor was hesitant to use this photo because he thought it looked more like an Ewok than it did a dog.

134 **This is known as "hypervigilance":** Hypervigilance in chronic pain patients is well documented. High levels of hypervigilance are common in pain sufferers and make pain worse. Rollman, Gary B. "Perspectives on hypervigilance." *Pain* 141 (2009): 183–184. McDermid, Ann J., Gary B. Rollman, and Glenn A. McCain. "Generalized hypervigilance in fibromyalgia: Evidence of perceptual amplification." *Pain* 66, no. 2–3 (1996): 133–144. Herbert, Matthew S., Burel R. Goodin, Samuel T. Pero IV, Jessica K. Schmidt, Adriana Sotolongo, Hailey W. Bulls, Toni L. Glover, et al. "Pain hypervigilance is associated with greater clinical pain severity and enhanced experimental pain sensitivity among adults with symptomatic knee osteoarthritis." *Annals of Behavioral Medicine* 48, no. 1 (2014): 50–60.

135 **Embracing positive sensations helps your brain feel safe:** Psychologists refer to the practice of leaning into positive sensations as "savoring." A recent study (in the awesomely named *Journal of Happiness Studies*) trained a group of students to use savoring in their everyday lives and found that it significantly reduced negative emotions like fear, thus making the brain feel safer. Hurley, Daniel B., and Paul Kwon. "Results of a study to increase savoring the moment: Differential impact on positive and negative outcomes." *Journal of Happiness Studies* 13, no. 4 (2012): 579–588.

In another study, chronic pain patients took an eight-week course that included savoring as one of its core components. After completing the course, the pain sufferers showed less pain hypervigilance. Garland, Eric L., and Matthew O. Howard. "Mindfulness-oriented recovery enhancement reduces pain attentional bias in chronic pain patients." *Psychotherapy and Psychosomatics* 82, no. 5 (2013): 311–318.

Chapter 9: Relapses, Resilience, and Recovery

142 **Bill Murray is stuck in a time loop:** *Groundhog Day*. Directed by Harold Ramis. United States: Columbia Pictures, 1993.

144 **My real dream was to be on** *Saturday Night Live*: *Saturday Night Live*. Created by Lorne Michaels. New York: National Broadcasting Company, 1975.

147 **"Even Jay Leno was terrible when he first started":** Jay Leno is famously self-deprecating about his early days in stand-up comedy. Leno, Jay. *Leading with My Chin*. New York: HarperCollins, 1996.

147 **Science has shown that you can become more resilient through practice:** Joyce, Sadhbh, Fiona Shand, Joseph Tighe, Steven J. Laurent, Richard A. Bryant, and Samuel B. Harvey. "Road to resilience: A systematic review and meta-analysis of resilience training programmes and interventions." *BMJ Open* 8, no. 6 (2018): e017858. Reyes, Andrew Thomas, Christopher A. Kearney, Hyunhwa Lee, Katrina Isla, and Jonica Estrada. "Interventions for posttraumatic stress with resilience as outcome: An integrative review." *Issues in Mental Health Nursing* 39, no. 2 (2018): 166–178. Parks, Acacia C., Allison L. Williams, Michele M. Tugade, Kara E. Hokes, Ryan D. Honomichl, and Ran D. Zilca. "Testing a scalable web and smartphone based intervention to improve depression, anxiety, and resilience: A randomized controlled trial." *International Journal of Wellbeing* 8, no. 2 (2018).

152 **a joke about his grandfather immigrating to America:** Just to bring things full circle, this Shelley Berman joke was retold by Lorne Michaels when he appeared on Jerry Seinfeld's web series *Comedians in Cars Getting Coffee*. Seinfeld, Jerry. *Comedians in Cars Getting Coffee*. Web series, July 14, 2016.

Postscript: The State of Healthcare and the Opioid Crisis

157 **patients did about the same whether they had surgery or not:** Mirza, Sohail K., and Richard A. Deyo. "Systematic review of randomized trials comparing lumbar fusion surgery to nonoperative care for treatment of chronic back pain." *Spine* 32, no. 7 (2007): 816–823.

157 **surgery had a much greater risk of complications:** This study found that the overall rate of complications from spinal fusion surgery was 11.5 percent: Faciszewski, Tom, Robert B. Winter, John E. Lonstein, Francis Denis, and Linda Johnson. "The surgical and medical perioperative complications of anterior spinal fusion surgery in the thoracic and lumbar spine in adults. A review of 1223 procedures." *Spine* 20, no. 14 (1995): 1592–1599.

This study (which also showed no benefits to spinal fusion surgery for back pain) found that 23 percent of patients who had this surgery had to have another spinal surgery within four years: Brox, Jens Ivar, Øystein P. Nygaard, Inger Holm, Anne Keller, Tor Ingebrigtsen, and Olav Reikerås. "Four-year follow-up of surgical versus non-surgical therapy for chronic low back pain." *Annals of the Rheumatic Diseases* 69, no. 9 (2010): 1643–1648.

157 **number of fusion surgeries in the United States actually went up:** Kolata, Gina. "Why 'useless' surgery is still popular." *New York Times*, August 4, 2016, A3.

158 **cost of chronic pain in the United States is more than $600 billion annually:** A report in *the Journal of Pain* estimated the cost of chronic pain is as high as $635 billion a year, which is more than the annual costs for cancer, heart disease, or diabetes. Gaskin, Darrell J., and Patrick Richard. "The economic costs of pain in the United States." *Journal of Pain* 13, no. 8 (2012): 715–724.

158 **buying every chronic pain sufferer in the country a new Rolex:** The Institute of Medicine found that a person suffering from moderate chronic pain generates $4,516 more in healthcare costs per year than a person without pain. For severe chronic pain, that number jumps to $7,726 per year! Pizzo, P., N. Clark, O. Carter-Pokras, Myra Christopher, John T. Farrar, Kenneth A. Follett, Margaret M. Heitkemper, et al. *Relieving pain in America: A blueprint for transforming prevention, care, education, and research.* Washington, DC: Institute of Medicine, 2011.

159 **more than 56 million Americans were prescribed some kind of opioid painkiller:** The CDC reports that in 2017 more than 17 percent of Americans had at least one opioid prescription filled. However, each patient received 3.4 prescriptions on average, so the total number of prescriptions was much higher. In the United States in 2017, the total number of opioid prescriptions was 191,146,822. These numbers are mind-boggling. *2018 annual surveillance report of drug-related risks and outcomes—United States.* Surveillance Special Report 2. Centers for Disease Control and Prevention, U.S. Department of Health and Human Services. August 31, 2018.

159 **Opioid overdoses are now the leading cause of accidental death:**
In 2017, 47,600 Americans died of an opioid overdose. That same year
in America, 39,773 people were killed by guns (including suicides),
and 40,100 died in car accidents. National Institute on Drug Abuse,
"Overdose Death Rates," January 29, 2019, https://www.drugabuse
.gov/related-topics/trends-statistics/overdose-death-rates. Mervosh,
Sarah. "Nearly 40,000 deaths from firearms in 2017." *New York Times*,
December 19, 2018, A19. Bomey, Nathan. "U.S. vehicle deaths topped
40,000 in 2017, National Safety Council estimates." *USA Today*,
February 15, 2018.

159 **life expectancy has actually gone down for the past three years:**
Saiidi, Uptin. "US life expectancy has been declining. Here's why."
CNBC, July 9, 2019. Retrieved from https://www.cnbc.com/2019/07
/09/us-life-expectancy-has-been-declining-heres-why.html.

159 **Centers for Disease Control has set new guidelines:** Bohnert, Amy
S. B., Gery P. Guy, and Jan L. Losby. "Opioid prescribing in the United
States before and after the Centers for Disease Control and
Prevention's 2016 opioid guideline." *Annals of Internal Medicine* 169,
no. 6 (2018): 367–375.

159 **a new fear:** that chronic pain patients like Brian won't be able to
get the opioids: Alltucker, Ken, and Jayne O'Donnell. "Pain patients
left in anguish by doctors 'terrified' of opioid addiction, despite CDC
change." *USA Today*, June 24, 2019.

160 **Eleven hours of pain content in the entire four-year curriculum:**
Estimates for pain education in U.S. medical schools range from nine to
eleven hours, with less than one hour specifically about opioids.
Greenfieldboyce, Nell. "How to teach future doctors about pain in the
midst of the opioid crisis." NPR, September 11, 2019. Retrieved from
https://www.npr.org/sections/health-shots/2019/09/11/756090847
/how-to-teach-future-doctors-about-pain-in-the-midst-of-the-opioid
-crisis. Shipton, Elspeth E., Frank Bate, Raymond Garrick, Carole
Steketee, Edward A. Shipton, and Eric J. Visser. "Systematic review of
pain medicine content, teaching, and assessment in medical school
curricula internationally." *Pain and Therapy* 7, no. 2 (2018): 139–161.

There are a few bright spots. A handful of medical schools, including
Johns Hopkins University and the University of Toronto, have added
multiple-day courses devoted to pain management and medicine to
their curricula. We need courses like these to become standard.

Index

Note: Page numbers in *italics* indicate photos.

negative thoughts
  as automatic, 126
  and believing messages of safety,
    130–31
  and catching your fears,
    126–30, 150
  weakening neural pathways of, 123
neglecting oneself, 125
neuroplastic pain
  about, 5–6
  as distinct disease, 161
  identifying, 28–29, 163–69
  mimicking of structurally caused
    pain, 169
  as most common cause of chronic
    pain, 6, 29–30, 56, 163
  onset of, 38–40
  origin of term, 28
  as real pain, 6–7, 10
  root of (see misinterpretation of
    signals by brain)
  treating (see Pain Reprocessing
    Therapy; the Process)
New England Journal of Medicine, 9
news, 107, 111
New Year's resolutions, 150
nucleus accumbens, 14

onset of pain
  associations between trigger and,
    54–55
  as opportunity to rewire brain, 96
opioid crisis, 158–59
outcome independence, 73–76, 143
overstimulation, 108–9, 149

pain-fear cycle
  addressing the fear in, 46
  author's experience with,
    43–44, 51
  breaking, with somatic tracking, 86
  distractions from, 58–59

fear's fueling of, 153
feedback loop in, 42–43
and gathering evidence for
  neuroplastic pain, 60–61
and perspective management, 96
and preoccupation with
  injuries, 140
safety as key to breaking, 154
Pain Psychology Center, Los
  Angeles, California, 1, 6
Pain Reprocessing Therapy
  and Boulder Back Pain Study,
    16–20, 29–30
  and breaking the pain-fear
    cycle, 46
  and Casey, 13–16
  conditions successfully treated
    with, 12
  development of, 6
  exposing the brain's mistake
    through, 65
  fostering a sense of safety, 47
  fundamentals of, 154
  as means of rewiring brain, 28
  and weakening neural pathways of
    fear, 123
  See also somatic tracking
panic attacks of Steve Martin, 53, 54
past events as source of fear/high
  alert, 36, 125, 166–67
patience, treating oneself with,
  124, 152
people-pleasing, 168
perception management, 51–52
perfectionism
  combating, with self-compassion,
    137–38, 152
  pressure generated by, 128
  as source of fear/high alert, 109
  as trait associated with
    neuroplastic pain, 167
personality traits associated with
  neuroplastic pain, 167–68
perspective management, 96

and somatic tracking, 67–68,
69–70, 75–76
when your pain is high, 91–92
Saturday Night Live, 144–45
Schubiner, Howard
and author's car wreck, 50, 51
and Boulder Back Pain Study, 16,
29–30
neuroplastic pain research of, x, xi
self-compassion
importance of, 124
patient's experience with, 125,
151–52
struggles with, 136–38
self-criticism
as source of fear/high alert, 38
struggling to overcome, 129–30
as trait associated with
neuroplastic pain, 167
sensitivity to pain, 109
setbacks
and building resilience,
146–47, 154
created by pushing through the
pain, 90
dealing with, 82–85
goal of minimizing, 88, 89
as normal part of the process, 89
when you have no pain, 94
when your pain is low, 109
short-term pain compared to chronic
pain, 15
Skinner, B. F., 98, 110
smart phones. *See* phones
social media, 107–8
somatic tracking, 65–78
breaking the pain-fear cycle
with, 86
and curiosity about pain
experience, 71, 72–73, 75–76, 77
duration of, 93, 101–2
exercise in, 70–72
frequency of, 93–94, 95
and "hawk mode," 72

importance of mindset in, 94, 95
intensity mitigation in, 72–73,
101–2, 143
mindfulness component of, 67, 69,
70–71
and outcome independence,
73–76, 143
patients' experiences with, 77, 101
positive affect component of,
68–69
role of language choices in, 77
safety reappraisal component of,
67–68, 69–70, 75–76
and sense of safety for brain, 149
and state of stress/fear, 141–42
used as weapon to fight pain, 101
when your pain is low or
moderate, 92–94
spinal fusion surgeries, 156–57, 160
stress
as automatic response, 114
family time as source of, 46
as form of fear, 44
onset of pain while experiencing,
29, 39, 61, 163–64, 165
patient's strategy for
regulating, 151
prevalence of, 106
and relapses, 140, 141
stress hormones, 107, 108, 110–11
structural causes of chronic pain
as assumed source of pain,
51–52, 136
biological instinct to link pain
with, 52–53
and biomedical model of
medicine, 55–56, 168
distinguishing neuroplastic pain
from, 28–29, 163–69
mimicked by neuroplastic
pain, 169
mistaken beliefs about, 153
neuroplastic pain as more common
than, 6, 29–30, 56, 163